Get a Life

Get a Life

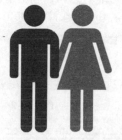

His & Hers
Survival Guide to
IVF

Richard Mackney & Rosie Bray

First published in Great Britain in 2015 by Orion
This edition published in Great Britain in 2017 by Orion
an imprint of the Orion Publishing Group Ltd

Carmelite House, 50 Victoria Embankment,
London EC4Y 0DZ

An Hachette UK Company

1 3 5 7 9 10 8 6 4 2

A CIP catalogue record for this book is available from
the British Library.

ISBN: 978 1 4091 5502 7

Printed in Great Britain by Clays Ltd

Every effort has been made to fulfil requirements with regard to
reproducing copyright material. The author and publisher will be
glad to rectify any omissions at the earliest opportunity.

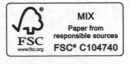

www.orionbooks.co.uk

To Molly, for making it all worthwhile.

Contents

Introduction   1

Foreword by Dr James Nicopoullos   5

Quick guide to the IVF process   7

Chapter 1   **What's wrong with us?**   8

Chapter 2   **Tests you will need**   22

Chapter 3   **How to choose a clinic**   42

Chapter 4   **Before your appointment**   62

Chapter 5   **Your first consultation**   82

Chapter 6   **The drugs**   99

Chapter 7   **Egg collection day**   116

Chapter 8   **Fertilisation results**   145

Chapter 9   **Embryo transfer**   162

Chapter 10   **The two-week wait**   178

Chapter 11   **Test day**   194

Chapter 12   **How to cope with a negative result**   208

Chapter 13   **How to cope with a positive result**   221

Chapter 14   **Diary of a miscarriage**   235

Chapter 15   **IVF finally works**   259

Chapter 16   **What we learnt from doing IVF**   281

Questions to ask at your consultation   293

List of terms   297

Acknowledgements   299

Index   301

Introduction

The first and most important thing to say is this:

DON'T PANIC

You will be surrounded by news stories and 'latest research' and newspaper and magazine articles and experts and people of your age with babies, all effectively telling you that you've left it too late.

But you haven't.

Because here's the good news: IVF works.

Not every time, and not for everyone, but it can and does.

That's why so many people are doing it now.

At the time of writing, 2 per cent of all babies born in the UK were conceived through IVF and around 50,000 women receive fertility treatment every year. IVF is now performed more frequently than well-known procedures such as having your tonsils removed.

And that leads us to the second important thing that we must say:

YOU ARE NOT ALONE

Whether it's down to financial worries, the pressures of the twenty-first-century lifestyle, bad luck or whatever, it doesn't matter; more and more people are using IVF because it offers hope and help.

That's why the fertility departments in hospitals are usually called 'assisted conception units'. Because that's what IVF is: assistance, a bit of help.

With this book we've tried to pass on everything we learned through three attempts at IVF.

Three very different attempts at three different clinics (including NHS and private) with three different outcomes: a complete no-show, a pregnancy and miscarriage and, finally, a successful pregnancy.

You will hear a lot of stories of people who did IVF several times before it finally worked.

But we believe, in line with that old cliché, that 'if we knew then what we know now' our first attempt at IVF would have had a better chance of working.

And we believe it could for lots of other people too.

What this book is for

One of the problems with IVF is that you are bombarded with an enormous amount of information, all of which seems important, but our aim with this book is to tell you what you actually need to know and what you don't.

We realised, by the third time we did IVF, that there was a lot of information that actually wasn't necessary and just caused us needless panic and stress.

We will, of course, explain the process and what happens at every stage along the way, but perhaps more important than that, we will also explain how you might feel at every juncture.

Because what fertility clinics don't tell you is how hard IVF can be on you emotionally and how it can severely test the most stable relationship.

That's why this book is a 'survival guide' and why each stage of it is divided into His and Hers. Even though you're going through it together, you'll each have very different experiences of IVF.

FOR HER

There's a breakdown of each stage, highlighting what you actually need to know and explaining how you might feel and how to survive every step of the process.

FOR HIM

We know from experience that men are often ignored during the whole IVF process, so there's advice on how to get through it, what you need to know, and how to deal with the trauma of wanking under duress. If you read no other sections in this book, Chapters 2 and 7 are essential...

How to use this book

Each of the His and Hers sections are generally divided into:

- **What actually happens**

  An explanation of what you will go through at each stage including fact boxes and stats.

- **What happened to us**

  Our personal experiences, including the emotional impact, the stuff we realised we didn't need to worry about, the stuff we wished we'd known more about and the mistakes we made.

- **How to survive this stage**

  Some tips at the end of each chapter, including key things to remember and advice on how to minimise the pressure and panic you may be feeling.

- **Where are you now?**

  Between each chapter there is a recap to remind you of where you are in the process and what's coming up next.

We have ensured as far as possible that all statistics and facts contained in the book are accurate and up to date, and for that we are hugely grateful for the help of **Mr James Nicopoullos,** fertility specialist at the Lister Fertility Clinic in London, who has gone through the book and checked our facts.

At the end of each chapter you will also find a section called **The Consultant Says;** here Mr Nicopoullos has added some of his own professional advice and tips to help you get through each stage.

Our aim is to help relieve the stress of IVF, to tell you what you will actually go through, how to deal with it and try to help you find a way to get through the process intact and with a successful outcome.

As you will probably know, IVF can be expensive and the odds are against you, but hopefully this survival guide will equip you with the best tools possible to save you time, stress and money.

We can't guarantee you will have a baby at the end of this book, but we promise we'll help you to survive the process.

Foreword

When we reach that point in life at which we decide we are ready to become parents, we are inevitably filled with a combination of excitement, expectation and perhaps a nervous apprehension at the huge responsibility that will soon be upon us. To make matters worse, this responsibility comes with no previous training or instruction manual!

It is against this background of expecting a positive new chapter in their lives that an increasing number of couples are faced with a struggle to conceive. The journey through testing, diagnosis and treatment with no guarantee of success at the end is an often turbulent rollercoaster ride that brings with it the kind of emotional distress that has been compared to the suffering of those diagnosed with a malignancy or experiencing a serious cardiac event.

At a time when you may feel powerless and lacking in the control that helps us all through difficult times, information is crucial. The emergence of the internet makes information more accessible than ever, but knowing what and who to believe and knowing how best to sift through the minefield of information for what is accurate and unbiased is just made harder.

This book provides couples with exactly what they need; an honest, accurate and invaluable portrayal of the highs and lows of their journey from start to finish, covering all the biology you need to know as well as the emotions and psychology that you should be prepared for. It is a book written for couples, by a couple.

In this book, Richard and Rosie have ensured that both men and women have the information they need and endeavour to provide them with the tools they need to cope with every step of the process. This is an essential read for all couples embarking on any fertility investigation or treatment and should be in every fertility clinic waiting room.

To have their trust and be asked to contribute, in even the small way in which I have, was a privilege.

James Nicopoullos BSc MBBS MD MRCOG DFFP
Consultant Gynaecologist & Specialist
in Reproductive Medicine
Lister Fertility Clinic

A quick guide to the IVF process

Just in case you don't know what actually happens with IVF, this is a typical cycle. (And don't worry, you'll hear plenty more about this process throughout this book.)

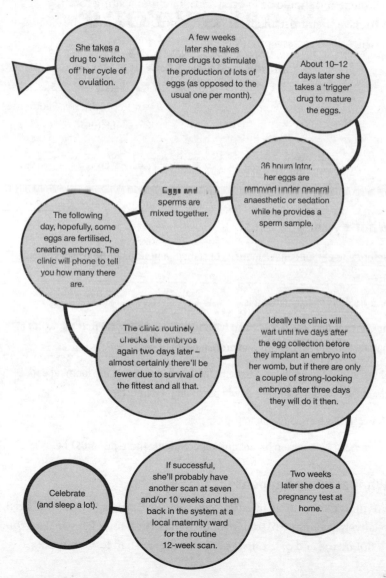

She takes a drug to 'switch off' her cycle of ovulation.

A few weeks later she takes more drugs to stimulate the production of lots of eggs (as opposed to the usual one per month).

About 10–12 days later she takes a 'trigger' drug to mature the eggs.

36 hours later, her eggs are removed under general anaesthetic or sedation while he provides a sperm sample.

Eggs and sperms are mixed together.

The following day, hopefully, some eggs are fertilised, creating embryos. The clinic will phone to tell you how many there are.

The clinic routinely checks the embryos again two days later – almost certainly there'll be fewer due to survival of the fittest and all that.

Ideally the clinic will wait until five days after the egg collection before they implant an embryo into her womb, but if there are only a couple of strong-looking embryos after three days they will do it then.

Two weeks later she does a pregnancy test at home.

If successful, she'll probably have another scan at seven and/or 10 weeks and then back in the system at a local maternity ward for the routine 12-week scan.

Celebrate (and sleep a lot).

1

What's wrong
with us?

HER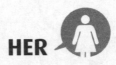

What's wrong with us?

Before you embark on IVF there is, of course, a period during which you are 'trying'.

And trying is exactly what it is.

Before that first discussion about IVF and visit to the GP, there is the world of natural fertility aids, charts and precision-timed sex.

There is also the underlying issue of fault and blame and the looming dark cloud that suggests you are slowly becoming 'an infertile'.

How can this be happening to us?

There must be a reason for not getting pregnant. There just MUST be...

What actually happens

We didn't start off as infertiles, we were just a normal, healthy (well, relatively), young (-ish) couple about to embark on some baby-making fun.

But by the end of the first year of 'trying' we had lost our spark.

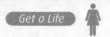

By the end of the second year sex had become very odd and was now laden with pressure, desperation and blame.

And by the end of the third year we had no choice but to accept that we had become 'infertiles'.

The Human Fertilisation and Embryology Authority (the statutory body that oversees IVF) defines infertility as 'a failure to conceive after regular unprotected sexual intercourse for one to two years'.

And it's more common than you might think.

How common is infertility?

- Fertility problems are estimated to affect one in seven heterosexual couples in the UK.

- About 84 out of every 100 couples who have regular unprotected sexual intercourse (i.e. every two to three days) will get pregnant within a year.

- About 92 out of 100 couples who are trying to get pregnant do so within two years.

Source: www.hfea.gov.uk/docs/HFEA_Fertility_Trends_and_Figures_2013.pdf

It was a slow descent into infertility – and it wasn't pretty. During that time we argued a lot about sex, parenthood, eggs, sperm and which of us was most likely to be the cause of the problem.

It will have been different for Richard, but the best way I can describe my 'infertility years' is that it felt as though I was existing under a little black cloud that followed me around everywhere I went.

Almost every day I would wake up and think, there's something bothering me, what is it? Oh yes, it's the fact that I don't have a child, or any prospect of having a child and I don't know if I'm going to have to rethink my whole life's purpose and the way I'd envisaged my future, and I have no idea when I am going to know this or if I will ever get over it.

Quite a big thought before you've even got in the shower.

Meanwhile, you are attempting to live a normal life where you congratulate friends on their pregnancies, their births, their second pregnancies – even their third in some cases. Chances are you're in your thirties and that's when pretty much everyone you know will embark on parenthood, so there's no escaping it.

And it's not just friends who are popping them out either. Suddenly it's everywhere you look – celebrities, people on the street, women on trains who you must give up your seat for whilst envying their rounded tummies and exhausted hot faces.

I realised my preoccupation was reaching pathological levels when I started skimming every interview I read with a woman, looking for her age, her children's age and working out how old she was when she had them. It's so innate in me now that I think I will always do it.

We'd obviously heard about the wonders of IVF but always thought it was for wealthy older couples, not for us.

In our minds it was the last resort – and an expensive one at that. Surely we wouldn't have to play that final card? Surely there would be a positive test result before then? Maybe this month I'd come up trumps? We've done everything we can think of to make it work, surely it will soon? But it didn't. And the pain and frustration and discord just grew and grew until finally we admitted defeat and started to talk about IVF – our great white hope.

It was quite a journey to IVF; this is how we got there.

Fertility facts

- Your body temperature rises after ovulation by up to one degree.
- You are most fertile on the two days before and on the day of ovulation.
- There is some evidence that female sperm lives longer; so if you want a boy, have sex as near to ovulation as possible, and if you want a girl, have sex up to four days before ovulation.
- One of the most accurate fertile signs is cervical mucus – when you see that becoming wet and slippery you should just get on and do the deed as it's the perfect place for sperm to live.

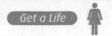

What happened to us

We got married. We threw away the condoms. We had fun. We were optimistic, excited even.

Then slowly but surely, months passed and there was nothing, except the familiar cramp of my monthly period, mocking me like a very punctual, very messy, uninvited house guest.

No problem. I am a natural-born researcher. I will take to the internet and find out what we can do about it.

Turns out there is endless advice out there.

Vitamins, diet advice, complementary medicine, stress relief and some 'scientific' failsafes.

Phew.

All is not lost then, we'll be fine if we just implement some of these new techniques and all that incredibly helpful advice that people dish out...

'Helpful' advice you will hear

- Stop worrying about it and it'll happen
- Just relax, maybe go on holiday
- Get really drunk and forget about it – then it's bound to happen
- Put your name on the adoption list – then you'll get pregnant naturally
- Eat more nuts
- Get a dog

My four-pronged approach

First, I invested in some **expensive vitamins** from the 'guru' of natural fertility, Zita West, then I bought a **fertility monitor** to measure ovulation and then I started **charting my temperature** every morning before getting out of bed (which is a right faff by the way). I also found a **hypnotherapist** who specialised in fertility and birth.

The theory was that the hypno would settle my mind, the vitamins would prime my body and then the monitor and thermometer would sort out when I was ovulating so that getting pregnant would become just a matter of time.

Well, that went on for a good year. And still nothing. By this point I'd given up on the pricey vitamins and reverted to bog-standard Pregnacare from Boots, had to up my hypno sessions to deal with the increasing stress of not getting pregnant and stopped taking my temperature every day. (My cycle was predictable enough and all I was doing was irritating Richard with the annoying beep of the digital thermometer at six o'clock every morning.)

I'd also done even more research and tried (and failed) to get Richard eating goji berries and walnuts for his sperm and I'd spent far too long examining my cervical mucus (whatever you do, don't Google it. Damn. Now I know that you will).

Precision sex

Now that I could fairly accurately pinpoint ovulation, we of course tried timing sex to fit.

Well, our exact routine actually started a few days before because (as I'd learnt by then) the sperm can survive in there for up to five days, although one to two days is more likely. Ideally you want them in there, swimming around and treading water, just before ovulation, ready and waiting, if you want the best chance of them meeting your lovely new egg and fertilising.

Richard didn't respond well to my incredibly unsexy and well-timed sex demands. And arguing about sex is surely the fastest way to create problems in the bedroom (which makes conception just a little bit tricky).

But the fun didn't end there every month...

Mind tricks

Each month we'd also go through the hope, phantom symptoms and absolute conviction that it had worked:

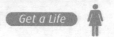

'I definitely did feel different this month, even a bit sick maybe. Yup, this is it, it's finally worked. I must be pregnant.'

It's amazing how you can be completely convinced and hopeful every month and still be surprised by the crushing disappointment of a negative test and the familiar cramp of an oncoming period. But it happened, every single month.

And when that period came, I would know I would have to get through a couple of days of proper gloom and sadness before the cycle would begin again and I'd be off on that same hopeful path to thinking that perhaps THIS month it would actually work.

With each period and each passing month the arguing and excuses increased, along with the desperation to find out what the hell was wrong with us.

Finally, when the months turned into years, we decided it was all getting a bit ridiculous. We'd given it a good enough go *'au naturel'* and now we just had to find out what the problem was. So, after a lot of delaying and deliberation, we decided to seek help from the medical profession and braced ourselves to take our tentative first steps towards IVF.

Success rates (pregnancies leading to live birth) for natural conception

Age when starting pregnancy attempt	30	35	40
	Success rate		
Conception within 12 months	75%	66%	45%
Monthly chance in Year 1	11%	8%	5%
Conception in Year 2	40%	35%	20%
Monthly chance in Year 2	5%	4%	2%
Total chance of conception within 4 years of starting	90%	84%	64%

Source: The Lister Clinic, London

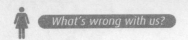

How to survive this stage

* Although you will know exactly when you are ovulating, try not to mention it to him. He will not care and he will just feel under pressure to perform.

* Have sex at other times in your cycle, not just when you know you're ovulating, so that sex doesn't become purely about getting pregnant.

* Do something for stress relief – hypnotherapy, yoga, aggressive spinning classes – whatever works for you.

* Don't put your life on hold. Although I loved it, I stopped running for three years as I thought it might damage a potential growing embryo that it turns out was never there.

* Don't tell people you think you really are pregnant this time; the more people you have to disappoint each month, the more disappointed you'll feel.

* Spare your emotions and your money and ditch the pregnancy tests. If you really are pregnant you'll find out soon enough.

* If it makes you jealous and angry, limit the amount of people you see who are pregnant or have newborn babies. If these women are friends, they'll understand you need to take a break for a while.

* Do stuff you can't do with children – go to the cinema, stay in spa hotels, eat in posh restaurants, stay in bed late...

* Be patient.

HIM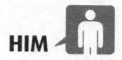

What's wrong with us?

In the absence of some glaring medical problem, before even considering the possibility of fertility treatment, you will probably go through these stages:

Having sex just like normal people ▻ having sex to try to get pregnant ▻ not getting pregnant ▻ her getting quite stressed about the whole thing ▻ him getting stressed about the whole thing ▻ being told exactly when to have sex ▻ getting even more stressed and being rubbish at sex ▻ her getting increasingly hysterical about sex ▻ him trying to avoid having sex ▻ arguing a lot ▻ realising it's time to get help

And bubbling away under all that ugly carnal discord will be the great unanswered question: what the hell is wrong with us?

What actually happens

Research has shown that one of the best ways to get pregnant is to have sexual intercourse. I know. Strange but true. According to scientists, that's what it was originally invented for.

But you will begin to notice that the sex you are having isn't really like the sex you had before.

Suddenly you're being told when to have it and sometimes you're tired or just not in the mood or in the middle of WHSmith.

Soon the sex needs to be had at a specific time on a specific day and you notice in your bathroom an increased number of complex-looking pieces of scientific equipment – gauges, timers, little plastic pens with small LCD screens – stuff so time sensitive they could predict unusual tectonic shifts, bank holiday weather or the exact migratory timetable of the crested water-thrush.

Now neither of you wants to have the sex at all and coital congress feels like the desperate, final hump of a pair of cancerous hippos.

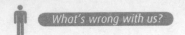
Both of you start to hate The Sex and excuses to avoid it that you never thought possible start to come out of your mouth.

Things you may hear yourself saying

- I've got a headache
- I'm too tired
- I'm really busy
- I feel really ill
- I've got the shits
- Surely we can just wait another month?
- I don't even want a baby
- I thought we'd already had sex today?
- I have no blood available for my penis
- I hate having sex with you
- I hate having sex
- I want to become a priest

With the arrival each month of the great menstrual Satan, The Scarlet Prince of Sanitary Towels, a little bit of hope dies and the tentacles of panic intensify their grip.

No other combination of five words becomes quite so unwelcome as 'I have started my period'.

Of course, there may actually be a reason, some traceable something to explain why she's not getting pregnant.

However, in the absence of previous problems or investigation, at this stage it's unlikely you'll know what's wrong.

It could be her. It could be you. It could be neither of you and instead just be, in that most unsatisfactory of English phrases, 'just one of those things'.

Conditions that may result in male infertility...

- Low sperm count
- Problems with the tubes carrying sperm
- Problems getting an erection
- Problems ejaculating

... And other factors

- Inflamed testes (orchitis)
- Past bacterial infection that caused blocked tubes
- Genetic problems
- Diabetes
- Lifestyle factors (like smoking, being overweight, etc.)
- Having a job that involves contact with chemicals or radiation
- Male fertility is also believed to decline with age

Source: HFEA

What happened to us

In fairness, my wife, Rosie, couldn't have been much more honest about wanting children.

I can remember an odd moment round about the third week after we'd first met, when she was still simply A Girl I'd Met At Work.

It was that baking summer of 2003, when mercury was rising in places you never thought possible, and when we were flirty and tanned, silly show-offs woozy on Pinot Grigio and hormones.

It was a 'just to let you know...' sentence, which I've learnt since means a point of vital information that should be logged and registered and never forgotten.

'Just to let you know, that if this does lead to anything long-term or serious I really do want kids at some stage.'

She was 27, I was 32.

'God, yeah, absolutely, so do I,' I lied, as part of a scheme by which I could have a proper go on her breasts.

The curse of thirtysomething
It wasn't really referenced or mentioned again until that monumental thirtieth birthday, that subtle difference, as someone once said, between £29.99 and £30.00. Suddenly you are No Longer In Your Twenties, you are now part of a group known as The Wrong Side Of Thirty.

Suddenly you are, well, old.

Now baby making is referred to with more regularity.

Now targets are being set: 'I want to have a baby by the time I'm 33', 'I'd definitely like to have two children before the age of 37', etc.

Fast-forward a couple of years and we find ourselves, entirely without warning, in a truly hideous, helpless parallel state known as Everyone Else Has Babies.

As a man, of course, you don't really care.

You feel almost nothing but pity for those friends who've had fatherhood thrust upon them. They disappear from view. If you see them at all they look and sound like they've died. They're exhausted and dull. Their faces are lined – they even smell grey. Whereas you still look the age you are.

The ever-ticking clock
But... you are going out with/married to/sharing a home with a biological creature for whom Other People Having Babies is like being stabbed in the soul.

This creature has had mothers, friends and almost every media outlet on Earth helpfully reminding her that her chances of having a baby are greatly reduced after the age of 35. She is fitted with apparatus that has a use-by date. It is non-negotiable and you will, with increasing regularity and force, be reminded of this.

Now it becomes a race.

You see and feel the urgency as your loved one spews out the fear of someone who's approaching exam time but hasn't done as much revision as her friends.

Her babied friends start disappearing too, of course, but where you feel nothing but a silent pity or superiority, she feels an all-consuming envy bordering on actual contempt.

Her babied friends now look ten years older than her, they are exhausted, saggy and pale, usually revoltingly ill, distracted, hopeless and boring. You tell her this but that reassurance means absolutely nothing to her; they have babies and she doesn't.

A thing called IVF

And so, after all of the above, over a period of about three years (the number of years IVF clinics and the NHS demand you must have been 'trying' to conceive), an increasingly internecine sex life, delaying the decision for as long as we can but with that body clock now DEAFENING, thumping out the soundtrack to our lives, we decide to pursue that thing that other people have tried and that apparently sometimes works. A thing called IVF.

The first stage is an appointment with the GP, and then it's time for one of the strangest wanks you will ever do.

How to survive this stage

* Having trouble conceiving when you need to is incredibly common. We are more stressed and older than previous generations so don't be alarmed if/when it happens to you. You are really not alone.

* Having said this, try to remember that this person you love is fitted with an entirely different operating system. She has an internal timer screaming at her to get pregnant.

* Be aware of strange behaviour. Aside from forcing you to mount her, she may start avoiding women and friends with babies. Anything that reminds her of what she doesn't have will hurt.

* She will be going through a type of hell, so be supportive. I know it sounds crass and weedy and I'll be saying that a lot in this book but, trust me, it makes life a lot easier.

* Don't be scared of reaching for the IVF card – it can work and just making that appointment with the GP will make you both feel you're moving in the right direction and may stop you killing each other or running off and becoming a monk.

The consultant says...

The journey to get pregnant is usually stressful enough. I think all the ovulation kits, the temperature monitoring, etc., turn things into a military operation which actually becomes counter-productive and increases the stress unnecessarily.

So rather than do those things, if you've got a regular cycle just try to have sex, mid-cycle, regularly and throughout the cycle. If it's still not happening, get some tests done sooner rather than later.

How quickly you seek advice will usually depend on your age. I would say don't leave it beyond a year if you're over 35.

Where are you now?

You have tried having sex (under increasing duress) but
she is not getting pregnant

*

Your bathroom cabinet has become filled with strange scientific
gadgets and charts

*

You are having sex only on the key days each month and
never for fun anymore

*

You are arguing a lot

*

You both realise something needs to be done

*

Time to make an appointment with your GP

2

Tests you will need

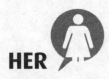

HER

Tests you will need

The very first thing to do after deciding that you need to get some fertility help is make an appointment with your GP.

The next thing you need to do is prepare yourself for a lot of tests.

Some of these will be simple blood tests, but others will have your legs in stirrups while a whole group of people in white coats 'umm' and 'ahh' at your vagina. Hopefully they will be medical professionals...

What links these tests is that they all could potentially indicate a mind-blowing problem – one that could mean you remain childless forever. Although this is unlikely, it does mean that even the most simple blood tests carry with them a nasty degree of fear and uncertainty and an unhealthy amount of time spent on Google.

You have to do these tests, though, if you want to get to the bottom of what could be wrong with you or your partner, so it's good to try to be systematic, positive and not get too hung up on the numbers.

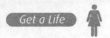

What actually happens

The most common blood tests ordered by the GP are:

FSH (follicle-stimulating hormone)

WHY? One of the most important hormones in the natural menstrual cycle, FSH is produced and released by the pituitary gland. It stimulates the ovaries to grow one or more follicles and ripen the egg within them. FSH also stimulates the ovaries to produce oestrogen.

LH (luteinising hormone)

WHY? LH is produced in the pituitary gland. A surge of this hormone during the middle of the menstrual cycle triggers ovulation (release of a ripened egg).

Estradiol (estrogen)

WHY? Estrogen is mainly produced by the ovaries and regulated by the pituitary gland in the brain. It causes eggs to mature and thickens the lining of the womb.

Progesterone

WHY? Progesterone thickens the womb lining to prepare for implantation of an embryo.

These tests will check that your hormones are balanced correctly and that you're ovulating.

Another blood test they may do is one that checks for German measles (rubella) which, if contracted during the first four months of pregnancy, can harm your unborn baby.

Your GP may also ask you to do a swab or urine test for chlamydia, which if left untreated can block your fallopian tubes, making it difficult to conceive.

They'll also issue a sperm test for your partner and possibly also a urine test for him for chlamydia, because it can also affect sperm function and male fertility.

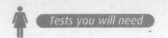

The results of these tests will determine whether there is some obvious problem or if you need further investigation at a fertility clinic.

What happened to us

Our blood and sperm tests didn't throw up any answers so we were sent for further investigations at a fertility clinic.

For us these were:

- A pelvic ultrasound scan to look at my uterus and ovaries.

- Hysterosalpingogram, which is an x-ray to check your fallopian tubes.

The pelvic ultrasound scan is an internal scan, so it's not like the films where they put jelly on your tummy and run a scanner over you while you smile delightfully at the screen.

For an internal scan they basically put a condom over a dildo, squirt some lubricant on the end and shove it up your vagina (albeit in as civilised and gentle a way as possible).

Although fairly undignified, this shouldn't actually hurt at all and it means they can have a good look at your uterus and ovaries.

If you are going to go on to do IVF you will have many more of these internal scans so it's good to get used to them if you can. Essentially, you need to leave all dignity and modesty at the door and think of this as just a little taster of what's to come.

The hysterosalpingogram, or HSG, was probably the test I disliked most, at least physically.

You have to be in the same position as you are during a cervical smear (i.e. clamped open), while they pass dye through your fallopian tubes and look at how it's passing through on an x-ray machine.

It can show (and clear) any blockages, and for many women just the act of clearing things out makes them able to conceive the following cycle. Sadly, this wasn't the case for us.

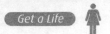
We could have opted for further tests, such as a laparoscopy (where dye is injected through your cervix as the pelvis is inspected via a telescope), or a hysteroscopy (a telescope with a camera attached to check for fibroids or polyps in your uterus), but I decided against it at that stage as these were both minor operations and it all felt too invasive.

My results

At this stage, before we ever attempted IVF, my hormone blood results were:

FSH   **6**
LH   **5**
Progesterone **33**

All these were deemed normal.

My pelvic ultrasound and HSG were also normal and showed no blockages or obvious problems.

Richard's sperm sample was average and we were both clear of chlamydia.

Our infertility diagnosis? Unexplained. Just like nearly a third of the UK population.

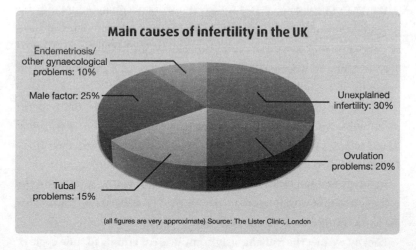

Main causes of infertility in the UK

Endemetriosis/other gynaecological problems: 10%
Male factor: 25%
Unexplained infertility: 30%
Ovulation problems: 20%
Tubal problems: 15%

(all figures are very approximate) Source: The Lister Clinic, London

The problem of the unexplainable

The thing about having an 'unexplained' diagnosis is that it's both good and bad.

Good because at least you haven't found a major insurmountable problem with either of you, but bad because at least if you had a medical problem then the doctors might have been able to fix it.

As it is you exist in this strange no-man's land where nothing is apparently wrong with you and yet you clearly still can't manage to conceive. You are really no further forward.

You start wondering if perhaps the problem isn't physical but mental:

- *Are you somehow jeopardising success yourself with some psychological block that needs sorting out?*

- *Should you be seeking holistic treatment or leave everything in the hands of scientists?*

- *Should you try to improve your nutrition or start a course of acupuncture?*

- *Should Richard stop cycling or talk to a hypnotherapist or eat loads of nuts?*

Being 'unexplained' basically means you're back to shooting in the dark. Great.

Yet being 'unexplained' also means there's still a glimmer of hope.

There's nothing actually wrong with you so in theory you still have as good a chance as any to conceive each month. Maybe you've just been unlucky all this time and there's still a chance it could all happen naturally.

Maybe the happy alchemy of the right egg and the right sperm meeting at the right time and implanting safely into your womb just hasn't happened yet. But that doesn't mean it won't. You still have hope and that's surely a good thing, isn't it…?

At 34 my body clock was ticking loudly and we were happy to be in the system, so our next step was to be put on the IVF waiting list. You will get used to waiting a lot at various stages during IVF.

Luckily we met the (ridiculously complicated) criteria for one cycle of

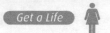

IVF on the NHS, but if we hadn't been eligible or if we had found out that the waiting list was really, really long, then we would have been looking at finding a private clinic.

How to survive this stage

* Stay off the internet. You are entering into a world of numbers and percentages and the possibilities of interpretation are endless and often unhelpful.

* Get the tests done as soon as possible. The sooner you get the ball rolling the sooner you will get on the IVF waiting list.

* Take the doctor's word for what is normal or not, try not to self-diagnose.

* When you're uncomfortable and sick of being poked and prodded, lie back and think of England (or Scotland or Wales or Ireland or, well, maybe just think of your unborn child).

* Even if you get a poor result on one of your tests, don't despair – modern science is pretty remarkable and it just means the doctors have more information to help you achieve a successful outcome.

* Resist the temptation to blame your partner if it turns out they are the one with a problem. It's not their fault and they need support, not accusations.

* Similarly, if it's an issue with you don't waste your time feeling guilty. At least you know what's going on now and can hopefully do something about it.

* Get organised. There is A LOT of paperwork that comes with IVF. Stay on top of all your appointments and file away your results. I sometimes felt as annoyed by the paperwork as I did by the drugs, so get control of it early on.

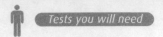
HIM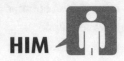

Tests you will need to have

Like most other medical balls, to get IVF rolling the very first stage is an appointment with your GP, who will need you to do a few tests.

If only they were basic arithmetic or word puzzles.

But they're not.

Your test will be to check the quality of your seed and *if you read nothing else in this book I'd quite violently recommend you read this bit and Chapter 7,* because IVF can test the resolve of even the most dedicated wanker.

What actually happens

The only condition to be satisfied at this first stage is that you have been 'trying' (that silly word again) for a baby for about two years.

Yes.

Of course you have.

Even if you haven't, you have. Two years is simply one of those arbitrary time periods that clinicians decide on at conferences and in scientific papers, so you may as well play along with them.

You may have been trying to conceive for much longer, or slightly less time; it doesn't matter, you will know by now that things aren't going well naturally and you need help.

As the gatekeeper to the world of medical expertise, the GP will explain that this first stage involves doing a load of tests, with the aim of trying to find out if there is any actual, traceable physical reason for your other half not getting pregnant.

Once the results are all in, and armed with all the fertility data about yourselves, it is then up to you whether you opt to do IVF or one of the 'lesser' fertility treatments explained in Chapter 5 – either funded by the NHS or funded by you.

But at this stage – like in the vast majority of fertility treatment – it is pretty clear that it is the woman who has the shittier end of the stick because pretty much all the tests must be done by her.

The first test, which is probably just a blood test at the GP's surgery, is to measure hormones, but the next round will be requested from a consultant at your nearest hospital.

The consultant will want to find out if all your lady's tubes and passages are operating properly, which will involve several unpleasant and, at times, painfully invasive examinations. For the full list, flip over to the 'Her' section of this chapter.

To be honest, you don't really need to know what these tests are called, just be aware that they're pretty nasty, intrusive and fairly emotionally draining. Even more so, of course, if the doctors find there is something physically wrong.

From the man, at this stage, the GP will simply require a sperm test. And that's how the GP will say it to you, simply a sperm test.

That's because they've probably never had to do one before. And if you haven't either, you need advice on this, my friend – trust me – as they won't give it to you.

The sperm test is a fairly unique form of humiliation, as you can see from the first-hand account (bad choice of phrase) in the 'What Happened To Us' section on page 31.

Sperm facts

- A low sperm count or poor sperm quality is the cause of infertility in about 25% of couples with fertility problems in the UK

- Up to 20% of young men find themselves with a low sperm count

- That means 80% of men have a normal sperm count, which means you probably don't need to worry

- The ideal temperature for sperm production is around 34.5°C, which is just below body temperature, so you need to keep those balls flapping around in loose clothing as much as possible.

- Vitamins said to help increase sperm count are: vitamin D, folic acid, selenium and zinc.

As I've said, at this stage the tests are a necessary part of the process of trying to find out if there is a definable reason for not getting pregnant.

Not unreasonably, I assumed the problem – well, that's what it is – lay with me. You will probably assume the same.

We're stressed, we're older than people used to be when they made families, we drink a lot and spend hours and hours staring at screens.

I naturally assumed my sperm count would be somewhere between insufficient and pathetic.

Lob in all those scary, fatalistic news articles that you will have also read about declining sperm counts in Western men and I assumed I'd have to take a load of vitamins, stop drinking and cycling, radically alter my diet or just have a full testicular transplant to get the numbers back up.

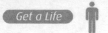

How to get the most from your seed

- Don't wank or have sex for at least two days before doing a sample
- But don't wait longer than ten days...
- Samples produced after two days of abstinence will have the highest numbers of good-looking, strong-swimming seed
- Try to get the sample to the clinic within one hour-ish
- Try to keep it at body temperature
- Try not to spill any

How you get your results

About a week after the deed, results are sent by post (sometimes you can phone and find out) – though sometimes I thought it would be nice if, like A-level results, they just put them on a big notice board outside the GP's surgery along with everyone else's.

I found it slightly terrifying opening that letter – like you're receiving the results telling you exactly how masculine you are. But what they check, why you have little reason to be worried and what the results actually mean is explained below.

What happened to us

The vessel

For your simple sperm test the GP will give you a small sterile plastic pot with a label on it.

Now, I am IN NO WAY the most well-endowed man within my local council boundaries, or even on my street, probably not even the most well-endowed man in my house, but I always found the little plastic pot just the teensiest bit small, almost spitefully small, just never quite big enough to make you feel confident that, well, you're going to get it all in.

The GP will also give you a form with your little plastic pot to confirm the sample is yours (presumably to eliminate the possibility that you'd be wanking off a friend and taking his spunk for him – I know, those horrible GPs trying to ruin a close friendship) and I think this is why on that form there is a question, underneath 'Name' and 'Address', that says 'Did you manage to get all the sample in the pot?'

Perhaps this is a little insight into the bored world of fertility doctors and it's a little bit of fun on their part, perhaps getting one up on you, the childless patient, because the answer almost certainly will be 'No'. It is impossible to get it all in unless the good Lord, in his strange and magical way, has endowed you with a pipette or fleshy calibrated dropper instead of a penis. And yet, nonetheless, you will almost certainly tick the box that says 'Yes'.

The deadline

There is also something a little cruel, I feel, about the opening times of the sperm-testing departments of NHS hospitals.

All the hospitals to which I've delivered sperm samples (and it now feels like I've hand-delivered seed to most of them in the Home Counties) insisted that I get my sample to them between 9 a.m. and 11 a.m. This might not sound too unreasonable, but the guiding rule is that they must receive the sample within an hour of deposit. In fact, 90 minutes is fine, they just want to be on the safe side. However, you probably don't live right next door to the hospital to which you have been assigned, even if it is your nearest.

That means you need to be transferring sperm from your testicular sac into your small plastic pot at around 9 a.m., and that means getting down to it fairly early in the morning.

That probably doesn't sound too bad – you may well normally do your wank at the crack of dawn, as it were – but masturbation on demand is a whole different type of masturbation.

I'm generally good with deadlines, and usually need them to get anything done, but wanking against the clock creates pressure and pressure for that delicate matter of self-abuse often isn't good. To properly understand the pitfalls, wait until Chapter 7, but for now just be aware that there is nothing normal or particularly pleasurable about masturbating under duress.

There's also the issue that watching porn at that time of the day seems somehow odd, even wrong. Perhaps it's just my paranoia but I'm convinced the 'actors' in the 'films' don't look like they're that into it at that time of day either.

The reason for the 'within-an-hour' rule is, of course, to keep your sample alive and at something close to body temperature. A couple of clinics to which I delivered my little pot of essence suggested putting it in a chest pocket to keep it warm, and one of them even suggested wrapping it in a sock.

Whatever you do, there is an indescribable feeling of oddness of being on a train, rushing to a hospital and realising you have about a hundred million tiny tadpole versions of yourself swimming around in your pocket. Well, hopefully in a sealed pot in your pocket rather than just loose, but you get the idea.

The shaky handwriting

Another top tip is that you need to write your name and date of birth on the label on the pot and I strongly advise doing this BEFORE your sorry act of forced self-pollution takes place.

Unfortunately my love of deadlines comes with my life-long battle with time-keeping and, maybe it's just me and how I do things, but it is always something of a rush to make that 11 a.m. closing-time deadline.

The first time I had to do a sperm sample, rather unsurprisingly, a little surplus did edge its way over the rim of the pot and I was in such a fluster to get out of my house and get it to the clinic that I temporarily lost the use of my right arm.

Such was the crazed and panicked intensity of producing my sample that my arm went into spasm and my name and date of birth became a few interconnected triangular shapes, more commonly seen on papyrus and legible only to scholars of ancient Aramaic.

The first time

That first ever sample needed to be at a hospital miles away. I didn't own a car but I knew it was a one-hour cycle journey, and so, as I scrawled my triangles on my smudged little pot, and attempted, with my non-spasmodic left arm, to seal the plastic lid I realised it was already 10.15 a.m. and I had 45 minutes to get there.

Not wishing to be turned back and to ever have to repeat this degrading process, my legs somehow raced my bike through a local park, slaying young lovers, joggers, and ambitious cottagers to get there. Suddenly it was 10.57 a.m. as I approached the hospital gates.

Unfortunately, I didn't factor in that hospitals are often quite big. And this one is big, really big, and rather cleverly I had managed to enter the gates on the opposite side of the hospital to where I needed to deliver my sperms.

I found somewhere to lock my bike – a caretaker's door handle – and looked at my watch: 11:02 a.m.

Panic. Real panic.

I ran through corridors, eventually asking a nurse where the hell the wing is that I need to be.

She thought about it.

Come on.

Please.

Christ's sake, hurry up.

Quick.

I need to know now.

'What's the rush?' she asked, hilariously. I said nothing, I couldn't answer her, I just pointed to my pocket and said, 'er, sample'. She looked at my swollen, twitching right arm and I think she understood.

Somehow I found the spunk desk. A dead-end bit of corridor with a few plastic chairs, no one waiting and a bored-looking woman behind a raised counter.

I explained that I was late and I had a sample and I was sorry I was late but please, please could she take it? She nodded, perfunctorily, took my transparent plastic bag and took out the pot and the form. She shook the pot slightly and held it up to the window. I have absolutely no idea why. What did she expect it to be?

'Um... it's sperm,' I said, unsure of whether she is a scholar of ancient Aramaic.

'Hmm' she replied, placed it next to her on the counter and smiled a smile of 'off you go now, sonny'.

I explained that I thought the clinic closed at 11 a.m. She asked 'what time is it now?' '11.08 a.m.,' I said. 'Oh God,' she replied, then darted out of her chair and through a door next to her clutching a hundred million tadpoles of me.

What I didn't realise is that if after all these preliminary tests you do opt for IVF treatment, the consultant will ask for more samples. They do love fresh sperm, these fertility specialists.

The second time

My second sample (this is still before we've even enjoyed our first attempt at IVF) needed to be at a different hospital.

By 11 a.m., of course.

I was late again, naturally, but I was learning from my mistakes. This time my name and date of birth were legible.

It was also a smaller building, a smaller affair, though in the sitcom of semen delivery, finding the department was easy, but finding the actual room to leave it rather less so. Just white corridors and no recognisable women behind counters looking ready to receive strangers' sperm.

I knocked on a few doors. Behind them there was no reply.

Eventually a woman who I assumed was a nurse popped her head round the corner and said I needed to go next door.

I went next door.

I knocked.

No answer.

Eventually I opened the door and two men in their mid-forties were sitting at separate desks. Both were on the telephone, both were well-fed and had beards. It felt like I had walked in on the 1970s if only the men were smoking too.

Neither looked up.

I stood in the doorway.

I am a polite, reserved man, not one to intrude. I was also a little shaky on this morning having masturbated against my will and against the clock and cycled three miles at a speed that can only be described as just under the speed of seed.

So I stood at the door and did that polite, simpering, expectant raised-eyebrows-smiley thing that only British people do. I did this for about a minute.

I looked at the time. It was 11.07 a.m.

My window had closed, I had a pot of slowly dying sperm in my pocket and two bearded men were inadvertently ruining my wife's chances of being a mother.

Eventually I got out my pot and held it in the air. I waved it a little.

Still the bearded men talked into phones and ignored me.

Eventually I approached one of the bearded men, brandished my pot and said 'Er, I've got some sperm'.

Beardy One looked up wearily. He points to the corner of the desk in a gesture that said 'just leave it there'.

I took it out of the envelope and – tempted as I was to unscrew the lid and smear the contents on his suit – put it on the corner of the desk.

I paused, expecting some kind of response, but Beardy One carried on chatting away as though strangers leaving pots of sperm on his desk was the most normal thing in the world.

I walked slowly out of the room and looked back a couple of times.

That's my son or daughter in there, you hairy-faced bollock, at least have the common sense and decency to pop him/her in the fridge or do something. But nothing.

Suddenly that 'within an hour' deadline they told me about seemed a little less urgent. Or perhaps it's just that the bearded men I encountered had no interest in expanding the population of their local borough.

Or – and it still crosses my mind to this day – I got the wrong room entirely and the Bearded Two were just bored account managers with a slightly warped sense of fun.

Results and what they mean

Despite yet more Shaky Hand Syndrome when I received the results letter a week or so later, to my surprised delight, my sperms were 'normal'.

Aside from delight, the other sensation was relief.

As outlined in the last chapter, in the world of fertility treatment there's a huge, all-pervading undercurrent known as 'Oh God, Please Make Sure It's Not Me'.

Whether blame is vocalised and discussed or not, have no fear, it is there, lurking underneath everything you do.

Every beer, every fag, every late night – and probably every wank.

'There has to be a reason for us not getting pregnant and it's probably you' is the ugly subtext.

Had my seed been sub-average, there would inevitably have been the mild barbs or spiky looks or even just a sense of withering hope every time I got another beer from the fridge or went cycling or did anything else that might, just might, be jeopardising my sperm-production facility.

Although, actually I imagine it's unlikely that even those rare men with super-seed are being cheered by their spouses or girlfriends when they pop open their sixth beer of the night.

Being average

On the results letter they don't describe your seed as 'normal'. Of course not. They say 'average' and then, when I thought about it for a moment, my delight dissipated.

Of course they were average.

There was no reason why they should be 94-carat, premier cru, elite super-athletes, the Phelps of the testicular pool, but equally there was no reason why they would be complete shambling wazzers.

Because that rather obvious realisation is a guiding principle to help to survive IVF: MOST PEOPLE ARE AVERAGE.

It's precisely what the term means. And it means that you probably are too. Which also means that statistically there will – almost certainly (that phrase again) – be no traceable reason for you not conceiving. Yup. It's just 'one of those things'.

Understanding your sperm test report

What they check	My results (from Dec 2010) – no, really	Normal ranges
Sperm count – the approximate total number of sperm cells present in your semen sample	255 million (Yes. 255 million. I mean, HELLO?? I could fertilise the whole of Scandinavia with that package)	More than 40 million
Sperm concentration – how many sperms per unit of volume	85 million per ml	More than 20 million per ml
Motility – how many of your sperms are actually swimming	60%	More than 40%
Volume – how much you actually produce	3 ml	2–8 ml
Morphology – how many of your sperms have a normal shape	35%	More than 30%
Viscosity – how thick or watery your semen is	Normal	Normal (ie. not low or high)

Normal ranges taken from our first semen analysis report

Of course, by the very law of averages, I may well have been one of the unfortunate minority of men who have a low sperm count. As I've learnt since, that MIGHT be down to lifestyle, or hobbies, or diet, but it might equally be none of these.

It might just be One Of Those Things and there are various ways to improve it and specialised IVF techniques to deal with it (see Chapter 5).

Equally, by the law of averages, the tests for your other half will (almost certainly) be completely normal, as they were for Rosie.

There is a greater number of variables that might not be functioning normally, and that's why she'll have more tests than you – and more unpleasant ones than your experience with your pot.

But almost certainly (sorry, that phrase again) there will be nothing to explain your infertility – as there wasn't with us – and this is a medical paradox. It's like going to the doctor with a stomach pain and the doctor doing lots of tests and being unable to find the cause of the pain. A bit of you actually WANTS him to find something wrong because then you'll know what exactly needs to be fixed.

Around a quarter of people who opt for fertility treatment tick a box marked 'unexplained'. And that's the box we ticked on every one of our three IVF attempts.

Maybe it's genes or age or stress or diet or lifestyle or environment, but it might equally be because of my taste in music or the socks I wear. It doesn't matter. The good thing for us was that there was nothing physically impeding pregnancy, which meant there was still hope.

How to survive this stage

* Get the GP appointment as soon as you feel ready – it's good to get the ball rolling quickly. After all, you can always cancel NHS appointments but at least you're in the system.

* Don't worry too much about the 'trying for two years' thing. It's a guideline. We were never probed on the issue. That was one of the few things that was left un-probed…

* The GP will describe it as 'just' a sperm sample, but if you've never done one before, leave enough time… If necessary, find out in advance where it needs to be delivered and what time to avoid bursting into the wrong offices with a pot of dying spunk.

* The whole 'getting the sample to us within an hour' is just a guideline. As near to an hour is better advice.

* Make sure you take it there in a pocket so that it's kept at body temperature.

* Don't worry too much about your sperm figures – your seed will probably be average, but if they are below average there are plenty of corrective measures that can be taken.

* Sperm quality/numbers has absolutely nothing to do with manliness or manhood or all that rubbish, so don't worry about it.

* And – a common theme in this book – these tests are much worse and more unpleasant for her, so try to bear that in mind and show a bit of spunk. As it were...

The consultant says...

My advice is to be a bit wary of the GP screening tests at this stage.

Unless there's something in your history that points to a particular problem, the most important test will always be assessing a woman's egg reserve because everything else is largely reversible or can be overcome.

However, the tests the GP does – FSH and LH, which are the initial markers of egg reserve – are generally not that accurate and can be falsely reassuring.

The AMH test is much more reliable but isn't usually done until a later stage.

Where are you now?

You have decided to get help

*

You have seen the GP

*

She has had blood tests and possibly scans

*

You may have had your first STD test for chlamydia

*

He has had his sperm tested

*

You now know whether it is a problem with her bits, his seed or
that frustrating diagnosis – 'unexplained'

*

Now it is time to decide where to get treatment

3

How to choose a clinic

HER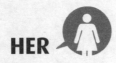

How to choose a clinic

If you are granted NHS funding you will be referred to a fertility clinic and may even have a choice of one or two to attend.

If you are going down the private route, there are hundreds of clinics to choose from and you need to do your research.

This chapter will tell you what to look for to help you make up your mind.

What actually happens

Whether or not the NHS covers the cost of your IVF treatment varies across the country and depends on your local clinical commissioning group (CCG) health board for your area.

IVF is currently pretty inconsistent across the UK; we've all heard of the IVF postcode lottery, so it's worth investigating what the rules are for your area via the HFEA website (www.hfea.gov.uk).

Will the NHS cover my costs?

In our case, we had to meet a long list of criteria to be eligible for funding, some of which are listed below:

- No more than two previous cycles of IVF/ICSI.

- Had to have been trying to conceive for at least 36 months or have a recognised cause of infertility (bizarrely, 'unexplained' counts as a cause).

- Had to each have a BMI of between 19–29 for at least six months before treatment.

- Must both be non-smokers for at least six months before treatment.

- FSH must be less than or equal to 11 iu/L.

- Must have blood tests done for HIV, Hep B and Hep C.

- Neither partner must have living children from this or previous relationships (including adopted children).

- Must be in a stable relationship.

- Must be under 40 when treatment begins.

- Neither of us must ever have undergone sterilisation before.

- Must be resident in the area of the CCG or health board at the time of treatment.

My particular favourite of these was the 'no living children' one.

I mean, I can understand why they say that, I get that funding is tight and they have to draw the line somewhere. But the fact that your partner may have had children years ago, even if they're nothing to do with you and not part of your life, would rule you out, does seem a little unfair.

And then it's just the terminology – a 'living child' just sounds so cold and brutal and gets you thinking about people who have been unlucky enough to have miscarriages, or worse.

It all points to a system where children have just become cold, hard facts and all emotions are going to have to go out the window.

Welcome to IVF.

What happened to us

In our area, the first time we did IVF we were only entitled to one NHS cycle of IVF (which we were extremely grateful for but, as you know, it failed) so for our second round we had to go private and set about finding a good clinic.

This is how we did it.

The fertility show

Luckily, just after our failed NHS cycle there was a fertility show on in London (held every year around November). We thought this would be a great opportunity to see lots of clinics and ask questions, etc.

It was useful, but fairly depressing too.

We went to some interesting talks by top fertility experts but the show was populated by endless 30-plus couples, with men being dragged around by women with a desperate look in their eyes.

I know we were no different, but it was pretty weird having a mirror held up to what we had now become.

We made ourselves feel better by making jokes about stalls with names like 'Fertility2U' and 'Fertility Astrology', not to mention picking up business cards from the European Sperm Bank that we could (hilariously) give to friends.

We got given a lot of leaflets and entered all the prize draws to win a free IVF cycle (I can't resist a competition) and Richard enjoyed chatting to the Spanish IVF clinic who were wooing passers by with wine and tapas. For a moment we thought some lovely holiday was on offer rather than months of injections and hospital procedures.

Meet the experts

The best bit about it, though, was being able to talk to top fertility consultants who you would never normally have access to (for less than around £200 per hour anyway).

We queued up to speak to one who was a bit like Father Christmas, granting an audience with each couple in turn for as long as they needed to go through all their questions.

We didn't actually go as far as sitting on his knee but we certainly felt like he was capable of granting our every wish as he calmly answered all our questions and reassured us that there was no reason we wouldn't be successful on another attempt.

We had already found a clinic that seemed good according to word of mouth and their online stats, and I'd also been to an open evening to hear a talk from one of their consultants, but meeting Santa and getting some advice and reassurance really helped to give an objective view.

After that we finally decided where to spend the £5K upwards that you have to expect to pay for a top clinic.

Despite ultimately being unsuccessful again, we were glad we chose that clinic for our second attempt, but it also taught us a few lessons about what was important when deciding where to go.

Key things to look for before choosing a clinic

1. **Location** – the nearer to you the better. You will have to go to your clinic A LOT. You'll have one or two initial consultations, numerous scans and blood tests and then of course the two main procedures (egg collection and embryo transfer) plus follow-up scans if you've been successful or follow-up consultations if you haven't. Weigh up the quality of clinic with its distance from your home and try to find a happy medium. You will not want a long drive or train journey when your aching ovaries are about to pop with maturing eggs.

2. **Cost** – check the brochure and ask questions about what is included. Some clinics may have a cheaper base price for IVF but expect you to pay each time for compulsory scans and blood tests, meaning it doesn't work out that cheap after all. Scrutinise the price menu as you would a budget airline flight booking – don't ignore the unexpected extras. A rough guideline from our experience is a final bill of £5,000–£7,000. This is a lot of money and even small savings can make a difference.

   Just to give you an idea, this is a range of a few of the prices charged for different treatments by the clinic we used in 2012:

Initial consultation	£260
Additional consultation	£130
IVF	£3,350
ICSI	£4,680
Ovulation induction and monitoring	£504

ADDITIONAL PROCEDURES	
Assisted hatching	£300
Blastocyst culture + Day 5/6 transfer	£560
Semen analysis	£140
Semen freezing and storage	£440
Semen storage per year	£300
Embryo freezing (1 year)	£600
Embryo storage (per year)	£300

3. **Drugs** – do you have to buy them from the clinic or are they flexible about you getting them elsewhere? Believe it or not Asda do fertility drugs (as well as some other companies who home deliver. I used 'Healthcare At Home') and they can work out substantially cheaper than your clinic's pharmacy. Yes, it may sound odd to ring up pharmacies and ask the going rate for human chorionic gonadotropin, but with IVF it really does pay to shop around.

4. **Stats/success rates** – most clinics will provide these or you can look them up on the HFEA website. Make sure you look at 'live birth' rates (a lovely phrase) for your age group as well as pregnancy rates to take into account the number of miscarriages the clinics produce. Also check their policy on multiple births. Most clinics prefer to aim for single births and so they limit the amount of embryos they put back unless you have exceptional circumstances. If this is something that concerns you and you want to try for twins, it's best to find out early on what the clinic's policy is.

Just to give you an idea, this is the national percentage of live births per IVF cycle:

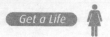

National live birth rate per IVF cycle started

Age	Live birth rate per cycle started
18-34	32.8%
35-37	27.3%
38-39	20.7%
40-42	13.1%
43 or over	4.4%

Source: www.hfea.gov.uk/docs/HFEA_Fertility_Trends_and_Figures_2013.pdf

5. **Word of mouth** – go on any of the fertility forums and you will find people discussing their experiences of clinics and consultants. From these, you can gauge which clinicians are considered good and have a reasonable bedside manner – believe me, there are plenty that don't.

   Better still, ask around any friends who've done IVF for their recommendations. It really is important that you find a consultant that you like. You are putting all your hopes and worries in their hands and you need to have faith that they know what they're doing and don't see you as just a number (although with the amount of patients they see at any one time, let's face it, you probably are).

6. **Flexibility** – what is their policy for when they do the procedures? Do they work bank holidays and weekends? Some clinics lump their procedures together to make it more convenient for the consultants, so for example they do all egg collections on a Monday or Wednesday and all embryo transfers on a Tuesday or Friday. But your body is growing eggs at its own pace (albeit spurred on by the nightly hormone injections) and may not fit in with your clinic's fixed dates, so you want to know how much flexibility they're prepared to give you.

7. **Clinic staff/nurses** – do you like their general attitude? You'll be dealing with them the most – you may only see the consultant a couple of times (and for one of those you'll be whacked out on general anesthetic) – whereas the nurses will become quite familiar faces.

You'll want to get a good feeling all round, from the reception staff booking in your scans to the nurses wielding their ultrasound probes up your skirt. You may prefer a cosy, homely approach or an efficient air of medical professionalism. Whatever your preference, speak to a few members of staff and see if they meet your expectations.

8. **Open evenings** – most clinics have these and they are a good chance to have a look around and also meet the consultants and find out their approach. I visited four clinics in total and they all had very different vibes. Some feel like hospitals, and are even situated in hospitals, whereas others feel more like your granny's living room or a sixth-form common room. Again, it depends what your expectations are and what environment you think you'll feel most relaxed in.

9. **Semen samples** – what facilities are available for men to produce their all-important semen samples? All clinics have private rooms for men to do their business but some better than others. Some have hatches where they can discreetly deposit (so to speak) their sample bottle when done whereas others involve walking it through a crowded waiting room to the lab technician behind reception. Some have state-of-the-art TVs loaded with porn options, whereas others rely on their trusty, crusty, jazz mags.

If you're not sure what your partner will put up with, best send him along for a quick look. Owing to the disaster on egg collection day during our first attempt at IVF (see Chapter 7) we needed Richard to be able to produce his sample at home and bring it in, which meant distance was a factor for us (they like to receive a sample within an hour). Some clinics might not let you produce at home at all, so it's best to check that out if you think your other half might have a problem producing under pressure on the day. According to the consultants we spoke to, that scenario is much more common than you might think.

10. **Instinct** – in the end, you can have researched all the facts and gathered all the stats but IVF is not an exact science (as all consultants admit) and until they know the magical contributing factor that leads to success or failure, it pays to be as comfortable as you possibly can be throughout the process. Perhaps it doesn't matter at all to the outcome if you feel tense or relaxed when you step through the clinic's door, or if you feel warmth or disdain from the staff – but just in case it does, why not listen to your gut and go with what feels good to you, even if that's not the clinic with THE highest outcomes. We're living proof that even going with what appeared to be an excellent clinic does not guarantee you'll be taking home a 'live baby' at the end of it.

A big step forward

Once you have settled on a clinic and have your first consultant appointment booked in, you will start to feel like you're making progress. You are now, at last, in the system and under the care of the experts, which will hopefully be reassuring.

You may also feel quite sad that you are definitely going down this route and having to have fertility treatment. You'll probably count how many natural cycles you have left just to see if a miracle could still happen.

In fact, lots of people will regale you with unhelpful tales of their friends who booked in for IVF and then just before they started the drugs, got pregnant naturally.

You, of course, still hold out hope that this will happen – and maybe it will – but it's best to make peace with the idea of IVF and even try to look forward to starting treatment. With a little (well, a lot) of luck you might just be pregnant in a matter of weeks. Hold that thought close to your heart and try to believe it.

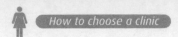

How to survive this stage

* Do as much research as you can using the sources described above.

* Remember that the clinics' stats are just stats. Try to visit a shortlist of a few clinics and get a feel for the places. In my experience, instinct had a lot to do with the decision.

* Bear in mind that you'll be paying the clinic a lot of money for treatment, so don't make a final decision until you are completely happy with it (the word 'happy' there is relative...)

* Try to view the experience positively (much easier said than done) – you are, after all, choosing the place which will hopefully result in you having a baby.

HIM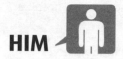

How to choose a clinic

It should be something of a luxury, choosing the place on the planet where you intend to conceive.

A chance, at last, to exert some control over the chaos as you elect the candidate you deem sufficiently competent to have the privilege of handling your essence and extending your family tree.

It should be an opportunity to leaf through glossy brochures assessing the quality of premises and the attractiveness of staff, to consider convenience and comfort before finally settling on the place where you intend to create new life.

Unfortunately, though, it's not really a luxury you will want or will necessarily have.

What actually happens

'Funding' is suddenly the ugly watchword.

If you satisfy the various criteria, the NHS will pay for the whole lovely experience for you.

You'll be sent a small selection of clinics/hospitals in your area. I say 'selection' but that obviously depends where you live and how many places in your area can actually do IVF. So the 'selection' may be just one clinic or it may be a few. If it is more than one you can choose which one.

If you don't satisfy the NHS criteria and you have to pay yourselves then, of course, you can choose where you want to do it. Anywhere in the country. Or abroad. This freedom to choose is only fair, really, given the hole it will leave in your bank account.

To find out how the NHS decides these things, have a look at the 'Her' section of this chapter on page 43.

This was our little history:

- First IVF attempt: NHS funded and given choice of three hospitals/clinics

- Second IVF attempt: self-funded and chose a clinic ourselves

- Third IVF attempt: NHS-funded again (as we had moved house to another area) and choice of two hospitals/clinics

When it came to choosing a clinic (from the NHS list or our own one during the second attempt), on all three occasions I generally left the choice to Rosie.

This is because when vital life-changing decisions come my way I have a clever coping mechanism which involves (a) hiding until they go away, (b) running in the opposite direction or (c) just passing them, buck-like, to her.

You may well do the same (well, not leave it to my wife, but leave it to your own partner) as they will have a far greater interest in the whole IVF process and will, by default, have absorbed lots of useful and useless information.

A lot of this will blow clean over you, but a few words of warning on where you will go to make your baby.

IVF clinics

- There are 78 licensed fertility clinics in the UK

- They do over 64,000 cycles of IVF each year

- Nearly 60% of these were privately funded

- Most clinics treat NHS and private patients so the level of care and treatment is the same, it just means that the NHS is picking up the bill

- The average cost of IVF is £6K per cycle and this can go up substantially if you need specialist services like ICSI (more on this later) or sperm donation, etc.

From The Human Fertilisation & Embryology Authority: 'Fertility Treatment in 2013: Trends and Figures: www.hfea.gov.uk/docs/HFEA_Fertility_Trends_and_Figures_2013.pdf

What happened to us

Choosing a clinic ourselves: word of mouth

After our failed, NHS-funded first attempt at IVF, when we realised that we couldn't get NHS funding for a second go and would have to pay for the whole thing somewhere ourselves, Rosie had – wisely or not – trawled websites and chat forums galore and had a fairly good idea of which clinics seemed good.

Suddenly, pregnancy rates and live birth stats were being bandied around like steeplechase odds, and often we rather forgot that what we were dealing with was the production of human beings, although in a way that gave new meaning to the term 'the human race'.

Much information was word-of-mouth, of course, from friends who'd done IVF and what their experience was like.

And that last bit is crucial...

Putting to one side all the physical factors of choosing a clinic, such as location and cost, and stats over how many live births are pumped out each year, how you are actually dealt with by fertility staff is probably THE most important factor.

Tiny asides, impatient remarks, overheard comments in corridors or just rude people in the wrong job can make or break the wafer-thin confidence of a woman undergoing fertility treatment. As a man you will feel largely ignored or patronised. You are a seed dispenser and that's all.

Some medical staff you deal with will be stressed or rushed or will have just had a bad morning or just won't have the necessary emotional tools for the task. And this stuff can't be taught or trained and isn't available in brochures or statistics.

Eventually, Rosie started taking down the names of specialists with whom friends of hers had had a helpful and pleasant experience (while obviously also bearing in mind how many actual babies they'd brought into the world) along with others she picked up from websites and forums. Very soon these names were being uttered in the same tone of voice as you would refer to minor gods.

There was even a chance to meet some of these baby-making gods before we chose a clinic for our second IVF attempt and to hear them speak out loud at an event in West London.

The fertility show

For two days in November, a large section of the Olympia exhibition hall becomes home to stands and displays and pamphlets as well as seminars and experts who want to fill your hearts with the possibility of childbirth and fill their bank accounts with the possibility of your money.

For our £11 entrance fee, we found ourselves wandering, bemused and childless, around the unborns' biggest trade fair.

The big names of the industry (well, that's what it quite clearly is and what this show is all about) were there, of course, like Zita West and Marilyn Glenville. But also there was stand after stand of clinics and companies you've never heard of, called things like Foresight, Serum and Vitro Life.

Expensive-looking men and women with immaculate teeth stood in front of brightly lit partition walls plastered with large, glossy photos of impossibly thin mothers triumphantly holding their impossibly healthy newborns in the air.

As we passed, each stallholder tried to suck in our custom, making us feel increasingly like not wanting to have a baby after all.

A long-haired man with long dirty fingernails leaped out and started selling his endemetriosis services to Rosie. He was, we were told, a 'world expert' on the subject. We had discovered, by the end of the day, that pretty much everyone at this trade show in West London was also a world expert.

After quite a lot of dirty-fingernailed questions about Rosie's vaginal bleeding, we tore ourselves (not literally) away.

Something for the gentleman

A tightly suited, shiny-haired Spanish man handed me a glass of red wine at one stand and gestured towards some plates of tapas. Well done, señor, for knowing how to attract the interest of men.

He showed us his thick-paged, glossy brochure with aerial shots of his fertility spa, olive groves and sun-parched hillsides and while I supped his wine and nibbled his chorizo he talked about the yoga sessions and hypnotherapy and nutra-lite tona-massage and aqua-sensitising aroma-toss and acu-nutra-hydro-wank, and by this time we were no longer listening, just standing entranced by the smoothness of this shiny man and his hair, silently adding him to a shortlist entitled 'Spaniards Who Are Unlikely To See My Wife's Vagina'.

An expensive moustache

Rosie had booked into some of the day's seminars, the first of which was by, surprise, surprise, a world expert on fertility.

A slim, smart, unassuming man, probably in his sixties, with a beautifully furnished moustache talked in front of a screen, his words illustrated by stats and pie charts and graphs.

I looked around the room at his packed, rapt audience; overwhelmingly female, hovering around 40 years of age and with sad, desperate eyes locked, unblinking, on the smart, slim man at the front of the room.

Every word, every syllable, every noise that came out of this man's mouth was devoured, as they stood there hoping beyond hopeless hope that he might make one sound, one tiny, barely audible utterance that will make them feel their childless years might be at an end.

I tapped Rosie on the arm.

'Look around the room – just look at them', I whispered.

'My God,' she replied. 'They're so old.'

Her face dropped. I knew what she was thinking.

They all looked so old. That meant that she thought she did too.

But she doesn't, because she's not. She's 35; it's just that the books and websites and newspaper features have told her she's left it all too late.

The power of percentages

The world expert spoke kindly but matter-of-factly, a surgeon with a good bedside manner.

He urged his audience not to get tied up in nutrition and fad diets, pointing out that women in Sudan and Ethiopia have plenty of children without all that rubbish.

His graphs and charts showed the chances of pregnancy in a healthy woman at different ages, percentages that become ever smaller after the age of 40.

The lines on the faces of the rest of the audience and the graphs made Rosie feel a bit better. But they made everyone there feel better, because even if a woman is told her chance of pregnancy at the age of 44 is just 2 per cent, it's still 2 per cent and not nothing. And there lies the curse of IVF.

IVF gives hope.

If you were in a casino and someone suggested putting seven grand on a 2 per cent chance of winning, it's rather unlikely that you would do it.

Whether it's wrong choices or bad choices, or bad biology or bad behaviour, or bad luck or repeatedly just being let down by bad men, at that point in that room with the smart man with the moustache going through his graphs, his whole audience heard what they wanted to hear because that man is an expert and he was saying he could get them pregnant.

Any questions?

Eventually all the graphs and data became too much and there was a shout from someone in the audience. A man was asking for help because his wife had passed out. The room was quickly cleared as first-aiders were bundled in.

But the world expert hadn't finished his presentation. And for the first time I believed that he wasn't just there to fatten his wallet. He said he'd continue in the foyer.

So all the sad eyes followed him out, not missing a sound or a gesture, and he carried on outside.

And he carried on.

And on.

The pack started to thin, but two hours later we were still there, two pairs of eyes among a group of about fifty.

Then he took questions. Dozens of them.

Women brought out folded pieces of paper with numbers and percentages on them and read them out to him and asked him what he thought and whether they still had a chance.

And the smart, slim world expert kept answering them, and he kept answering until finally Rosie said we could go and we left the world expert in the smouldering centre of the flickering hopes of about 20 sad-eyed childless women, fully expecting him to be there until the following March.

Weeds

We went to another seminar, where we listened to a Chinese woman who told us which herbs we should take to get pregnant. Yes. At last. The herbs.

That was what had been lacking from these middle-aged, childless women, they hadn't had any extortionately priced sachets of dried weeds from these people. Even Rosie, who had paid to be sat there, was affronted and decided we could finally leave.

An audience with Santa

But before we finally escaped the spunk circus, Rosie wanted to go to the stand of one of the clinics to get some more information.

But we couldn't actually get there.

There was a queue of women and couples – about 20 of them. We peered round to see that at the end of the queue, perched on a stool, was the exhausted-looking world expert with the moustache who was still talking to anyone for as long as they wanted to talk, the fertility version of a grotto where Santa was emptying his plump sack of embryos to those who'd been particularly good that year.

I couldn't take it any more.

We turned towards the exit, I swiped a pile of calling cards from the International Sperm Bank, something to remember the day by and perhaps send anonymously to friends, my final memory being me pushing through another crowd of desperate, sad-eyed women overflowing from the Astrology Fertility stand – yes, really, Astrology Fertility – before we finally exited the Dark Ages to get a very twenty-first-century sandwich.

* * *

The cost

Of course, having had our first attempt funded by the NHS, the world of costs when choosing a clinic ourselves was all new to us.

In the end, after our trip to the Fertility Show and with her research skills and vested interest being far greater than mine, Rosie settled on the clinic where we would make our self-funded second attempt at IVF. This delighted me as I didn't have the patience (or, to be honest, the desire) to scour online brochures and live birth stats and, ultimately, she would be the one who needed to feel comfortable at the fertility clinic that would be treating her.

You will probably be the same way – but if you do want to have more say, have a look at the Her section of this chapter for all the key factors that are useful when choosing a clinic. They generally hold 'open evenings' where you can go along and get a feel for the place and the staff, though I would say that location is pretty important.

There is also the small matter of cost.

Notice above that I say 'Rosie settled on the clinic', though the 'settling on' was greatly helped by the bottomless hearts of Rosie's parents, who dug into their savings to help out.

Generally, very broadly, the cost of IVF at the moment in the UK is around £5,000–£7,000. I say around as there are also various 'lesser' IVF options, covered in Chapter 5.

And, as I've mentioned, the total cost should cover everything, including the most punitive charges, which tend to be for all the scans and blood tests and all the drugs.

We didn't have a spare £7,000 sloshing around in our bank accounts – you may well be the same – so cost is, unfortunately, also a massive consideration.

Going overseas

There are also other options available abroad. One friend of mine discovered that you could get a three-for-one offer in Copenhagen and spent around seven grand and two years trying to get pregnant there, but that's pretty much my sum knowledge of the overseas experience.

Although I do now know a place in the Spanish hills where you can get a hydro-wank and free tapas...

How to survive this stage

* If you knew nothing about IVF before this you probably at least knew that it was expensive. Getting NHS funding could save you around £7,000 but it is governed by that postcode lottery which is just unfair and that's that.

* If you do get it covered by the NHS, remember to factor in NHS waiting times.

* If you don't get funding, leave the choice of clinic up to her, as where you have your treatment is as much about the right 'feel' of the place as it as about their success rates – and women are just better at that stuff.

* Check for 'hidden' costs, like blood tests, etc.

* Go to a fertility show if you want to actually meet a consultant and get face-to-face advice, but try to avoid astrologers, oily Spaniards and men with dirty fingernails who want to go up your wife's vagina. Actually, I try to live my life by that rule.

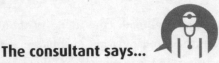

The consultant says...

There are going to be a number of clinics in your location that will give you a very similar chance of getting the outcome you want.

The most important thing is feeling comfortable in a clinic and having confidence in the people that you are seeing.

Visit clinics, go to an open evening, have a chat with one of the consultants and get a feel for the place.

Success rates are of course important, but you have to feel comfortable wherever you are being treated.

Where are you now?

You decided to get help

*

You have now started the whole process

*

You have seen the GP and got your test results

*

You know whether you can get NHS funding or not

*

If you got funding, you will have been allocated a clinic, a consultant and an appointment time

*

If you didn't get funding, you have researched and chosen your clinic and booked in to see them

*

Now a bit of advice before that first appointment...

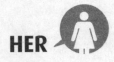

4

Before your appointment

HER

Before your appointment

Whether you've lucked out with the NHS or you are paying through the nose from your own funds, you've waited a long time to see your IVF consultant and no doubt been through a lot both mentally and physically beforehand. You'd better make it count.

These consultants charge hundreds of pounds an hour and you want to get your money's worth.

So, you need to go prepared and with a list. Yes, a list.

Your partner might hate you for looking like a demented control freak but just ignore him, this is all too important.

This chapter will help you decide what you need to ask, including things we wished we'd asked before we embarked on our first IVF attempt.

We'll also cover the pre-consultation tests you will be asked to have – including HIV and the dreaded AMH: two acronyms loaded with emotion.

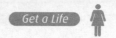
What actually happens

A few weeks before you meet The Consultant (aka the miracle worker, saviour of sanity, the godstar who is going to solve all your problems and change your status in this world), you usually meet a nurse.

The paperwork

Meeting the nurse is not quite as exciting as meeting the consultant, and what usually happens first is that you have to go through an awful lot of paperwork – pages and pages of questions. Be aware, too, the questions are pretty legalistic and pretty crude:

USING EGGS AND EMBRYOS FOR RESEARCH AND TRAINING

Do you consent to your eggs being used for training purposes?
YES/NO

Do you consent to embryos (already created in vitro with your eggs) being used for training purposes? YES/NO

IN THE EVENT OF DEATH OR MENTAL INCAPACITY

Do you consent to your eggs being used for training purposes?
   If you die? YES/NO
   If you become mentally incapacitated? YES/NO

Do you consent to embryos (already created in vitro with your eggs) being used for training purposes?
Please note that embryos can only be used if the sperm provider has also given his consent
   If you die? YES/NO
   If you become mentally incapacitated? YES/NO

Other uses for your eggs and embryos

If you wish your eggs or embryos to be used for the treatment of others, please complete as relevant:

• Your consent to the use and storage of your donated eggs (WD form)

- Your consent to the use of your donated embryos (ED form)
- Your consent to the use and storage of your eggs or embryos for surrogacy (WSG form)

However, if you do not give your consent in this section or on one of the forms mentioned above, the eggs or embryos must be allowed to perish in the event of your death or mental incapacity.

(Form taken from: www.hfea.gov.uk/docs/HFEA_MT_form.pdf)

A good (or boring) half hour is spent ticking boxes like 'in the event of Richard's death...' and affirming that you have never been to prison or been in trouble with the police.

As I've said before, nothing is sacred or deemed private when it comes to IVF.

You also have to make decisions about things you really know nothing about at this stage – like whether you'll be happy to donate any leftover embryos to research once you've completed your family.

The idea of completing your family is so alien to you right now that you can't possibly imagine how you are going to feel about tiny specks of you floating around in saline solution in five years' time.

More tests

As well as tedious paperwork there are also some extra tests to be done at this point. The nurse will want you to be tested for:

- chlamydia (always for the woman, if you haven't already, and sometimes for the man)
- hepatitis (B and C)
- HIV

What happened to us

Having an HIV test felt like quite a big deal to us.

As kids of the eighties, we both well remember the 'Don't Die of

Ignorance' campaign that was pretty terrifying to an 11-year-old.

Those images of a 'deadly disease', hammering letters on to a giant tombstone coming crashing down to earth, are indelibly marked on our memories. Scary stuff. And well done to the 1987 public health office at the time because the disproportionate fear and hysteria that followed that campaign stayed with all of us well into the nineties and our university days.

As unlikely as it was, not knowing if you had HIV (or rather full-blown AIDS because really that was what it was all about) was one of those scary daydreams you occasionally let yourself have.

We all knew it could take ten years or longer to develop, so maybe that drunken fumble with that Canadian with the white socks during freshers' week or the frightful encounters with the dirty lothario next door had actually marked your card forever and were set to ruin your life all these years later. It was enough to send shivers down your spine.

So it was with some trepidation that we both went for our HIV tests.

It was at least a welcome distraction from the IVF and we both started to get nervous about receiving a phone call asking us to come in and 'discuss the results'. No one wants to hear that.

But luckily that didn't happen and the results were (as any sane person would have predicted) completely clear. That was an unnecessarily happy day and worthy of disproportionate celebration: 'I'm clear, I'm alive, I don't have AIDS! Hooray!'

Ridiculous.

The dreaded AMH test

The other test that I had to have was to affect me so greatly that it blasted the HIV test into oblivion. And this time I had no preparation for the consequences at all.

But just so that you don't have this thrust upon you with no warning, let me tell you all about the dreaded AMH test.

AMH stands for anti-müllerian hormone.

Some clever spark in a lab somewhere discovered that measuring the level of this hormone in your blood can give a fairly accurate indication of how fertile you are – that is, how many eggs you have left – in terms of quantity and quality (generally the theory is that the more eggs you have the more likely it is that you will have some good-quality ones among them).

This measure of your fertility always used to be done by testing your level of FSH (follicle-stimulating hormone) and LH (luteinising hormone). If your FSH was high, it indicated that the brain was having to produce more FSH to work the ovaries harder to make one of the eggs grow each month ready for ovulation.

But FSH tends to fluctuate quite a lot within a month and from month to month. The level was taken at the beginning of the menstrual cycle and, as it is produced by the brain to act on the ovary, it is not a direct measure of the egg reserve in the ovary so sometimes throws up misleading results.

This is where the AMH test comes into its own – the level stays the same throughout the month and tends not to fluctuate from month to month so it is considered a more stable measure of fertility than just looking at FSH alone.

Having always had all my tests come back normal – including my FSH – I had come to terms with our fertility diagnosis being 'unexplained' and so fully expected this simple blood test to come back reassuringly average as well.

So it was a huge shock to hear that I had pretty low AMH – a number of 6.4 to be exact – which put me in the low-fertility bracket.

AMH levels explained

- Optimal fertility: 40.04–67.9
- Satisfactory fertility: 21.98–40.03
- Low fertility: 3.08–21.97
- Very low/undetectable: 0.0–3.07

Aaarrrgh!!

So there it was in black and white:

LOW FERTILITY

I was officially running out of eggs (as if I didn't know that already from reading newspaper scare stories every week).

Being a suspicious type, I asked to get the test repeated (which was met with a disapproving sigh as it was explained to me that the test results don't fluctuate). But I insisted and had another blood test two weeks after the first.

This time the results came back a bit higher, 9.2 (it turns out that AMH results shouldn't fluctuate but can within the bounds of lab error), but I was still in the low fertility bracket so the doctors were not that interested in the minor fluctuation.

However, no one explained that those average AMH levels in the box above are for all ages so they also include all those buxom, fertile 16-year-olds who are bursting with lovely fresh eggs, as well as the dried-up old hags like me.

Thankfully, one clinic I found provided an alternative chart showing average AMH levels per age group, which made for slightly less hysterical reading.

Average AMH by age

AGE	AVERAGE AMH LEVEL
25	24
30	17.5
35	10
40	5
45	2.5

www.ivf.org.uk/media/54656/How-is-ovarian-reserve-assessed.pdf

Why they do the AMH test

They like you to do an AMH test before embarking on IVF because it is said to give doctors a good indication of how you'll respond to the drugs.

For example, if you have a low AMH like me, the doctors will put you on a high dose of stimulating drugs as the theory is you'll need a lot of help to push those few remaining eggs out.

If you have a high AMH, this could indicate either very good fertility or, at the other end of the scale, potential polycystic ovaries. If that is the case the doctors will want to give you a low dose of stimulating drugs so that you don't push out a ridiculously high number of eggs which can cause serious problems and pose a health risk.

Therefore I reluctantly accept that it is a useful test to do.

The fact that I always produced good numbers of eggs (between 8 and 13) and once produced 27 eggs (well above what they aim for or what is considered normal) means I don't know how accurate this correlation is, but it is what doctors now use to help them decide on drug dosage.

Ignorance really is bliss

I found the AMH test a deeply distressing part of the process and wonder if it would be better if the doctors just did it secretly and didn't involve the patient in the results.

Knowing my score meant that I freaked out even more about my declining fertility and sent myself into a panic about my time running out and being a childless, wizened old lady.

It may well be helpful for IVF doctors, but I think it is rarely helpful for the patient to have an actual score put against their fertility reserves. Especially as this is a relatively new test that has been used increasingly over the last decade and there are some studies that show it can be affected by factors such as low vitamin D.

Some women get a score of less than one. How desperate does that make them feel?

And yet, even so, these same women can be successful with IVF (and even naturally) and go on to have children. In my opinion the AMH test

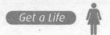

opens a can of worms and I wish it could be avoided, but at the moment it is what the IVF doctors focus on.

You can, of course, ask for the figure not to be disclosed and I would strongly recommend that you do.

The main thing is, if you get an upsetting result, try to remember that it's just the latest and most fashionable test and there'll be a new one along soon. Also, you only need one good egg. That's a cliché you'll hear a lot, but it's true.

Questions you need to ask at the consultation

Tests done, results gathered, you're nearly ready for your first consultation with The Doctor (High Priest of Babies, Captain Embryo, Wizard of Fertility, Knight of the Round Tummy, etc., etc.). But remember, your time with them is precious (and also costing about £4.20 a minute if you are paying) so these are the key things you need to ask.

To save you copying them all down, these questions are repeated on pages at the back of the book so you can just tear them out and take them with you.

1. **What drugs will I be on?**

   (Required for down-regulation, stimulation and triggering the release of the eggs – there is a more detailed explanation of all these in the next chapter.)
   - What dose will I be on and why?
   - How do I administer the drugs – are they all by injection or do I sniff the down-regulation drug?
   - When will I be shown how to mix up and inject the drugs?
   - Can I source the drugs myself or must I buy them from your pharmacy?

2. **What is the timeline?**
   - How soon can I start?
   - On what day of my cycle do I start the down-regulation drugs and how long am I on them for?

- When is my baseline scan to assess that all is shut down and quiet? When will I start taking the stimulating drugs and how long (on average) after stimulating is the egg collection?

3. How often will I have monitoring scans/blood tests?

(Not all clinics do blood tests.)

- How flexible are the scanning appointments (i.e., Do you have many early morning appointments so I don't have to take time off work?)
- What size follicles do you look for before deciding when egg collection should be?
- How many eggs are you trying to get for me at egg collection (given my age, history and test results)?

4. Where do you do egg collection?

- On site or elsewhere?
- Who will do the procedure? You or a colleague? (Most consultants share patients so you won't necessarily have met them before the op.)
- Will I have general anaesthesia or sedation?
- What pain relief will I have after egg collection?
- How long will I need off work after egg collection?

5. When and where is the sperm sample produced?

- Can we see the room beforehand and can my partner do a test sample to check he's comfortable there?
- Can we freeze sperm as a backup? (All clinics should offer this.)
- If so, how much does this cost?
- Can he bring in a sample from home instead?
- When should he do his last ejaculation before THE sample that is to be used?

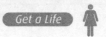
6. **Where is embryo transfer carried out?**
   - How many days after egg collection do you prefer to do egg transfer? (Most clinics have a preference for two-, three- or five-day transfer – this is properly explained in Chapter 9.)
   - What is your view on three-day (eight-cell) transfer versus five-day blastocyst transfer? (Also explained in Chapter 9.)
   - What is your policy on single embryo transfer v multiple (for our age and circumstances)?
   - What are the risks of a multiple pregnancy?
   - How do you grade the embryos? (Some clinics have different grading systems.)
   - Will you try to freeze any spare embryos?

7. **How do you rate our chances of success given our age, history and test results?**
   - Is there anything we should do (exercise, acupuncture, diet, supplements, etc.) to increase our chances of a successful IVF cycle with you? (Some clinics advocate acupuncture or total bed rest after transfer, etc.)

8. **What are the risks involved with the procedures (OHSS, etc.) and also any side-effects of the drugs?**

9. **In what circumstances would you decide to abandon the cycle?**
   - How common is that and at what stages do things go wrong?
   - If it didn't work, when would we be able to try IVF again and what support would there be from the clinic?

10. **How much does it all cost?**
    - Are the scans/blood tests all included in the base price or are they on top?
    - How much are the drugs on top (given my particular dosage) and what about follow-up consultations (if unsuccessful)?

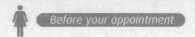

How to survive this stage

* Easy for me to say now, but try not to read too much into your AMH result. It created a whirlwind of panic in me that was completely unnecessary.

* If you prefer, you can ask for the AMH result to be withheld.

* Don't worry too much about the other tests – it's unlikely you'll have chlamydia or HIV, despite 1980s' public health campaigns.

* Try not to drown in all the paperwork – get some box files and get organised. I once had a meltdown over all the bits of paper I had over my three cycles and it really is not worth getting stressed about.

* **TAKE THAT LIST OF QUESTIONS WITH YOU**. They are repeated at the back of the book so just tear out the pages and take them with you. It may seem ridiculously anal but it will prevent that moment when you get home when you think, 'Oh shit, I forgot to ask them about...'

HIM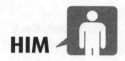

Before your appointment

Yes, I know this is an overblown title for a chapter that implies you need to do hundreds of hours of late-night revision and buy a special outfit.

In fact, it's just a few things to think about before you see the specialist – things we didn't ask the first time and wished we had.

What actually happens

Box ticking

Before you have your first consultation with a specialist (who really is viewed like a minor deity concealing beneath their cloak the wonderful gift of life, hitherto denied you), you'll probably have an appointment with a nurse.

This is just administrative, making sure that every box has been ticked before you embark on your IVF journey, but be aware there are A LOT of boxes to tick.

There will be forms to fill in that cover every eventuality: whether you will want to freeze 'spare' embryos, and for how long, whether you want to keep any frozen sperm and for how long (yes, of course there's a charge for this), what should happen to the embryo in the event of your death or mental incapacity, whether you want to submit the outcome of your IVF results to aid research, etc., etc.

This is boring and time-consuming and really used to annoy me, but then I'd take a step back and remember what this was all about and that if it takes a lot of form-filling to borrow money to buy a house then it should really take quite a lot of bits of paper, time and admin to make a human.

More blood tests

The nurse will also ask for yet more blood tests to be done before you see the specialist so that the results are as recent as possible. They can probably be done at your GP's surgery and include hepatitis B and C, chlamydia and AIDS. And don't worry – you probably haven't got any of them.

To freeze or not to freeze

One thing you should consider at this stage is whether to freeze a sample of your sperm. Yes, I know it's a weird thing to consider and it conjures up all kinds of images of sci-fi and cryogenics, but have a read of Chapter 7 and you'll understand why it's quite a good idea.

Freezing sperm can relieve a lot of the pressure of egg collection day (THE key day in the IVF cycle). There is obviously an extra cost to do this, though, so ask the specialist how much it is and when you could do it.

If you do decide to do this there will be more consent forms (every legal eventuality needs to be covered, remember?), but it's fairly standard stuff:

- What will happen to your sperm should you become unable to make decisions for yourself or die.

- How long you want to store your sperm (the standard storage period is ten years).

- Whether your partner (if you have one) can use the sperm later to create a family and whether you wish to be recorded as the father of any child born as a result of fertility treatment after your death.

- Whether your sperm can be used in research or donated for use in someone else's treatment.

- Any other conditions you may have for the use of your sperm.

> ## Frozen sperm facts
>
> - Sperm is frozen in liquid nitrogen.
> - Some sperm do not survive or are damaged during freezing. This means that after freezing there may be a reduction in quality.
> - There are no risks to patients (or children) from using frozen sperm.
> - Sperm cells have been frozen and thawed successfully for more than 40 years.
>
> (from www.hfea.gov.uk/74.html)

What happened to us

Three terrible letters

As you will have gathered already, IVF largely consists of percentage chances and acronyms. You will hear loads of mostly three-letter abbreviations during the process.

They mostly don't concern you as they all affect her, and I could never remember which was which, but there's one you really should know about.

These three letters created untold panic in our formerly happy household and sent us stampeding towards the IVF departure gate when perhaps we could have been a little more rational and considered.

The three letters are **AMH.**

I don't really know what the AMH test actually is – and you won't need to either – other than it is a blood test for the woman that is done at this stage.

It's another number that fertility clinics need/like to have among the long list of other numbers to give the specialist an overview of most appropriate treatment.

But I do know that whoever told Rosie the detail of her AMH test result was directly responsible for releasing into her head the exact sentence that would make the remainder of her thirties a fast-running egg-timer of paranoia, fear and despair.

An unhelpful thing to say to a childless woman

AMH is a blood test that ultimately measures how many eggs a woman has left until age renders her infertile. That means it's a number that, theoretically, shows how long she has left before she's infertile.

Now, what I now know about IVF is that probably THE worst thing you can possibly say to a childless woman in her early thirties or older who has been looking forward to having a child for the majority of her time on earth is 'you've got a low number of eggs and you'd better get a move on'.

Rosie had her AMH test, not really knowing or thinking about the implications, and was told, very matter-of-factly that it was 'quite low and she should probably try IVF sooner rather than later'.

That statement was enough to ruin her day, her month and the next four years.

Which means it ruined mine too.

And that means it could ruin yours.

She had, in so many words, been told to hurry up and that the odds were rapidly against her, that she didn't have many eggs left, that she'd be infertile soon, that her chances of conception were dwindling faster than those of a normal woman of her age, that time was very much not on her side, that she'd actually left all this a bit late, that she probably would end up childless and that the rest of life would be silent, unbearable and pointless.

The needless panic

From the clinics' perspective, AMH is a pretty invaluable tool as it gives a fairly accurate measurement of a woman's egg reserve.

However, if/when your partner is told she needs to have the test, also make sure you have the discussion about whether you want to know the result. You have a right to say that you don't want to be told it and it can be kept discreet among medical staff, never imparted, as a guideline to add to all the other factors on their list.

That may be the most sensible decision, because for us that AMH number induced panic, and panic is the great enemy of IVF.

Remember: you are only a man

As well as all the paperwork this is also your first chance to feel useless.

The nurse will, almost certainly, be female and, almost certainly, will barely look at you or address you directly.

Remember that you are just a spunk dispenser and have no feelings or empathy or useful input, in fact, you have nothing whatsoever to contribute.

This used to annoy the crap out of me, but you will get used to it. The important thing you need to know to survive this stage and not get furious and throw things is what to ask about when you do see the specialist – which will probably be a couple of weeks later.

The important bit

If you flip over to this same section in the 'Her' side of this chapter you'll see a long list of questions. They will probably mean nothing to you as they don't concern you, which, in fairness, is why men are so overlooked at this stage.

However, it is vital that you find out from the consultant EXACTLY WHAT YOU WILL HAVE TO DO ON EGG COLLECTION DAY – the culmination of the month-long IVF process.

At our first ever appointment with the specialist, during our first IVF cycle, when I asked what I would have to do, particularly at the culmination of the whole process – egg collection day – I was politely batted away.

'You've got the easy job', 'All you need to do is turn up on the day and do your business'. Etc., etc.

It was obviously all a piece of piss and I laughed it off like a feeble Englishman, feeling almost guilty for asking. Lucky old me. I've got the easy job.

Horseshit. Total horseshit. If you want to skip ahead and find out the actual, sordid details of your 'easy job' then read Chapter 7. For now, though, make sure you get satisfactory answers to these questions when you eventually have the consultation with the specialist.

If necessary, write them down and take them with you so everything is covered, or just tear this page out and take it with you. This stuff is important.

Don't allow yourself to be ignored or dismissed, even jokingly.

It's what we believe contributed to the failure of our first IVF attempt.

What you need to find out

1. What actually happens on egg collection day?

For the man, egg collection day is the most important day of the IVF process. For one month your lady partner will have been taking lots of drugs to stimulate egg production. The egg collection day is when she goes into the hospital/clinic and, under general anaesthetic or sedation, has her eggs removed and put into an incubator. You must then produce a sperm sample within an hour or so of this happening.

2. Can I freeze a sperm sample a few weeks before egg collection day?

This takes away a lot of the psychological pressure you might experience when you have to produce a sperm sample on the day. Just wanking into a pot sounds straightforward – after all, you've got the easy job (yeah, right) – but actually, ejaculation in a noisy booth surrounded by several other grunting wankers under the strict pressure of a time limit can do odd things to a man's mind and libido.

Also, it turns out that, just like peas, frozen is as good as fresh, it is only the defrosting process that kills sperm – about 50 per cent of it – but the rest is fine.

3. If you're paying for your treatment – and even if you're not – find out if you can give another sample to be frozen if the first one isn't good enough.

They should let you know the quality of your sample (motility, and the actual number of the little buggers) to make sure it's within their parameters. But if you have to do another one, find out if you are being charged – and if you are, find out how much it will be.

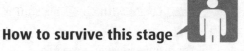

How to survive this stage

* Be patient with all the paperwork. There are loads of forms to fill in but remember that you're trying to create a human, so it's fair enough.

* Remember that stuff about AMH. It's a massive shitter for a woman to know. It's effectively setting the stopwatch. Try to make her not panic. (Yup, good luck...)

* Even better, discuss with her whether to ask the clinic to keep the AMH figure to themselves. You can demand this and it might save A LOT of unnecessary worry.

* Don't laugh at her huge list of questions to ask. I know it will seem obsessive and mad but specialists are busy and expensive people and this is a rare chance to find out EXACTLY what you need to. This could mean the difference between IVF working the first time or having to do it again, as we had to.

* Find out about the egg collection day – skip forward to Chapter 7 if you need to know why. And do not let them dismiss you with 'you've got the easy job' rubbish. If they do, perhaps ask them how many times they've had to reach orgasm in a booth against a strict time limit, armed with a very well-thumbed, crispy old jazz mag and surrounded by noisy wankers. That should shut them up.

The consultant says...

Before your appointment, it's important to do a little bit of research.

BUT... beware of Dr Internet because a lot of the information that's out there online is inaccurate and can make you perceive that your chances are going to be very, very small when in fact they're often better than you anticipate.

Basically, you need to have done enough research to know what you need to ask, but just don't believe everything that you read.

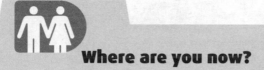

Where are you now?

You know where you're doing your IVF treatment

*

You have seen a nurse at the clinic

*

You have done the remaining blood tests

*

You probably haven't got AIDS

*

You have made a long list of questions to ask

*

You have come to terms with the idea of fertility treatment

*

Now it is time to meet the consultant who will hopefully make a baby for you

5

Your first consultation

HER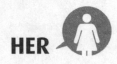

Your first consultation

At your first consultation you will be given a timeline of how IVF should go.

A lovely, simple timeline that takes you from A (infertile) to B (pregnant).

God, that sounds good.

But it rarely is that simple, so this is your opportunity to quiz, probe and generally annoy your doctor by asking about all the variables along the way.

What actually happens

It's quite exciting going to this first ever consultation on your first foray into IVF.

We were full of nervous expectation, hoping that this was the beginning of a process bringing us one step closer to having a baby.

It was nice to feel you were actually doing something and making progress, and about to meet the clever genius doctors who were going to make it all happen with their special instruments and fine art of drug mixing.

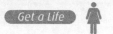

Of course, by the time we were on our third round of IVF, quite a lot of this optimism had dissipated and our initial meetings with consultants went very differently, but the first one was definitely a mixture of hope, excitement and confidence.

How your bits work

The first time we did IVF, we met a nice lady doctor who went through all the basic information we needed to know via a complex doodling technique:

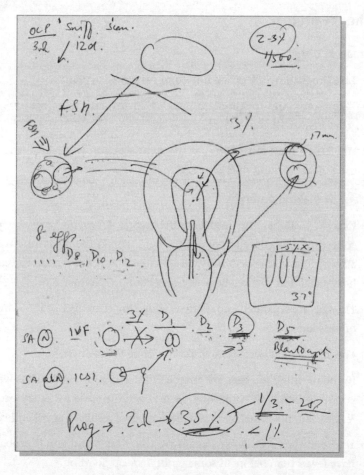

She drew a fairly rudimentary GCSE replica of the female reproductive system and from there, using lots of arrows and numbers, explained the risks, odds and likely outcomes of achieving a 'live birth'.

For my age group (35–37) at this clinic, this turned out to be about 30 per cent, which is pretty average in the UK.

Anyway, let me take you through the basic step-by-step IVF process (the drugs are covered in detail in the next chapter). I've broken it up into four stages as it's quite a lot of info to take in.

The IVF process

Stage 1: Drugs

• Take drugs to switch off your natural system of ovulation.

• Take more drugs to stimulate lots of follicles (and therefore eggs) to grow, instead of your monthly one egg.

• When you have lots of eggs at the right size you will take a 'trigger' drug to mature and ripen the eggs.

Stage 2: Making embryos

• Exactly 36 hours after you take the trigger drug you have the 'egg collection' procedure to harvest the eggs. This is the most invasive of all your procedures and is usually done under general anaesthesia or heavy sedation. (More about egg collection in Chapter 7.)

• The eggs are separated and sperm is added (by either IVF or ICSI – more on this later).

• The eggs are left overnight while you hope for the best.

• In the morning the eggs are checked for fertilisation and this is when your numbers start to decline, as it is very unusual for every egg to fertilise. But now you have a certain number of fertilised eggs = embryos.

• Your embryos are checked again two days later and you'll probably have fewer than before as some embryos stop dividing.

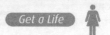

- Hopefully you'll still have some embryos left that are still dividing and looking good. This is where it all comes down to maths and odds.

Stage 3: Putting embryos into your womb

- The doctors want to put back the best embryo (or embryos; in the UK it is a maximum of two unless you are over 40), so they need to be able to pick which ones are doing the best in terms of division and also fragmentation (which seems to mean how unevenly edged they are). Again, it all comes down to numbers.

- So, if on Day 3 you have two clear embryos that look better than the rest, it's worth getting those two back inside you ASAP. The theory is that as long as you can tell which embryos are your best bet, they will do better in the womb than in the lab. This process is called embryo transfer and is a bit like having a smear test (see Chapter 9).

  However, if you have five good-looking embryos that all look like they're progressing at the same pace, it's impossible to tell which one is the best. So you might take a gamble and wait until Day 5 to put one back.

- By Day 5 another one or two (but hopefully not all five) embryos will have started to lag behind and there should emerge one or two clear winners which you can then put back. Leaving them until Day 5 means the embryo is now called a 'blastocyst' – basically it has divided hundreds of times and, rather than dividing cells, it now consists of two masses, one of which will become the placenta and the other the fetus. At least one blastocyst is what everyone is aiming for because they are strong embryos that have withstood the process so far.

- Doctors are happy to put back two Day-3 embryos but are much more reluctant to put back two blastocysts, the theory being that by Day 3 the embryos still have a way to go and the chances are that both probably won't carry on dividing and make it into a baby. But with a blastocyst the embryos have proved themselves to be much stronger by surviving to that point, so there is more chance of them both continuing and therefore increasing the risk of twins.

- There's also a risk of further multiples, as embryos can sometimes divide to make identical twins, and sometimes even triplets. So you could put back two embryos on Day 3 and end up with six children! This is extremely unlikely but it is, in theory, physically possible.

- Once you've had embryo transfer on either Day 3 or Day 5, your lab will still keep an eye on any remaining embryos to see if they continue to divide. If any look good and make it to blastocyst by Day 6, they can freeze them (if you wish) to keep for future use – either if this cycle fails or for a sibling to your new baby.

Stage 4: The wait...

- The final drug you will take is progesterone (either injections or suppositories – nice) and you take that from egg collection day until you do a pregnancy test. If negative you then stop taking it, but if positive you continue taking it for a period of time. How long differs depending on your clinic, but often it is until you reach that all-important 12-week milestone.

- At 14 days after your egg collection (regardless of when you did your transfer) you will do a pregnancy test at home and learn the outcome of all this effort and physical and emotional upheaval.

So that's the timeline of events, but of course each cycle of IVF comes with a million different what ifs, worries and pitfalls.

It all sounds so straightforward when written in a list like that but, as anyone doing IVF will tell you, it rarely is.

Fairly common complications

- You can respond strangely to the drugs.
- You can have odd complications during the monitoring scans (like cysts).
- You could have follicles without eggs or immature eggs or overcooked eggs and then you might have zero fertilisation once the sperm has mixed in.
- Your embryos could start behaving strangely and dividing slowly or not at all and you might be left with nothing to put back.

And then of course there's absolutely no guarantee you'll get pregnant, even with two perfect-looking embryos; your body could still mess it all up and for some reason not allow them to implant.

You will be warned of all of this at your consultation, but hopefully you can ignore all the doom-mongering and assume everything will be as straightforward as the timeline they'll give you.

It's a real testament to the power of IVF that you'll place all your hopes and dreams and the best part of anywhere between £5k and £10k on about a 30 per cent chance.

Surely with odds like that the only sensible thing to do would be to back a safer bet, but unfortunately with IVF (at least with your own eggs/sperm) you are usually taking a rather large gamble.

It was only at our third consultation that the doctor admitted there is so much they don't know about the whole process and that someday they will probably know much more about why things go wrong – sometimes even when everything looks to be following the textbook scenario.

And that is the problem with IVF. It's a risky business.

Your ART (artificial reproductive techniques) options

During your first consultation you will no doubt discuss all your treatment options, depending on your individual results.

For example, if it looks like there is an issue with your eggs then they'll probably suggest straightforward IVF, but if it looks like there is a sperm problem they may go straight for ICSI. And then of course there's IUI – a cheaper alternative and often the first port of call for the infertile couple.

IUI: You take a lower dose of a stimulating hormone drug to boost your follicle development and when your follicles look good the semen sample is washed so that the best sperm are injected into the uterus. Then you wait 14 days to do a pregnancy test.

IVF: As explained on page 7.

ICSI: The doctors look under a high-quality microscope for the best-looking sperm they can find, then they pick it up and inject it directly into the egg to sort of force fertilisation. This procedure is generally used when there are problems with the sperm – either they're not moving fast enough or there are a lot of damaged ones with malformations.

IVF, for all its drugs and science, generally follows the principle of natural selection, i.e. the egg is surrounded by millions of sperm and then left so that the strongest and best sperm wins the quest to fertilise the egg.

ICSI, however, bypasses natural selection and some people think it is therefore a bit more controversial. Scientifically, it means that although doctors can choose a good-looking sperm they have no way of knowing if it really is the 'best' sperm of the bunch and they are still only going by looks alone. There is no way of seeing if a sperm carries DNA damage – only that if it looks good it is more likely to have good DNA.

So, sometimes ICSI embryos are considered a bit less robust in the early stages, though by the time they've reached blastocyst stage you can be pretty sure they are strong.

There is also some controversy over ICSI babies, as one study showed there were some genetic defects carried from fathers to sons via ICSI, but these were generally the low-sperm problems that had led to the father seeking ICSI in the first place.

IMSI: ICSI with a more advanced microscope. This method is more expensive and a little more effective at picking out the best sperm of the bunch.

Donor eggs, donor sperm and donor embryos: If you already know your eggs or sperm are shot (or if you're in a same-sex relationship) you may opt for a donor option to either make up the other half of the puzzle or go straight for a donor embryo which has already proved to be a strong contender.

It is very rare and expensive to find that donor embryos, donor eggs or sperm are more commonly available. One consultant told us during an open day how helpful it would be in busting the myth that you can be fertile well past the age of 40 if there were a celebrity donor egg mum who would actually speak up about it.

There will be waiting lists and prices for donor eggs and sperm and you can decide what you want in terms of eye colour and hair colour, job, etc. – a bit like shopping for a pizza but less tasty.

Egg sharing: If you are under 35 (and reach some other criteria like a normal AMH and FSH) and are paying for your treatment, your clinic might offer you egg sharing. This means that they expect you to produce quite a few eggs so that you can donate half to a stranger and drastically cut the costs of your treatment, often only having to pay the HFEA licence fee of £75 and the cost of ICSI, if needed.

What happened to us

Hopefully your first consultation won't have been too overwhelming and will have filled you with excitement and hope rather than doubt and despair.

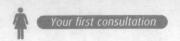

Just one thing to note, though, whereas *you* will feel armed with information and equipped with knowledge, your other half will probably feel a bit affronted.

In most of our consultations Richard was treated as an afterthought, only gifted a vague glance when sperm was mentioned.

One doctor actually dismissed one of Richard's questions with a joke, telling him that he had the 'easy job to do'. No real thought was given to how he must be feeling or what he should know about the process.

IVF is all about the woman.

And that short-sighted attitude is what can spark off a huge psychological block that can lead to your entire IVF cycle being wasted, as it was in our first attempt.

So be warned, do not underestimate the benefits of a good consultant who treats you both as partners in this process. After all, as we've always been told, it takes two to tango (or make a baby at least).

How to survive this stage

* Take a notebook. Your doctor will be telling you all sorts of information that you will not remember but that you will want to digest properly later.

* Ask questions. Take in that list from the last chapter if you need it. This is your only chance to cover everything so don't leave anything out.

* Don't be embarrassed. It can feel a bit strange to be discussing something so intimate in such medical detail but the consultants are more than used to it and will happily discuss sperm for as long as you want to.

* Be truthful. They need to know if you've had an abortion or sexually transmitted diseases before. They are not going to pass judgement. Full disclosure is key.

* Get the doctor or a nurse to show you how to do the injections – it's complicated and you need to be fully confident that you can do it.

* Take your time – don't feel rushed. These consultants see hundreds of first-timers like you every month; you may feel like you're burdening them with all your questions, but this is your moment and this is important, so take as long as you need. They won't chuck you out.

* Give your partner the opportunity to ask any questions that he has – everything will have been directed at you but the man's role is just as important and you want him to feel confident and involved too.

* Make sure you come out of there knowing what your drug protocol will be (and why) and when you can start.

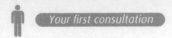

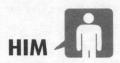

HIM

Your first consultation

This is the first appointment with the specialist, who will probably be the same one who oversees your IVF process.

They will explain how the process works, what to expect, and how long it all actually takes.

And remember, whether they are a man or a woman, you will be largely ignored, so just be ready for that and remain calm.

What actually happens?

The important bit

Up until this stage you will probably have just been showing a passing interest in IVF, mostly to avoid arguments and to appear all nice and supportive to your partner.

But before you go into that first consultation with the specialist, it's quite helpful to know the basics of the IVF process.

The IVF process

- She takes a drug to 'switch off' her cycle of ovulation.
- A few weeks later she takes more drugs to stimulate the production of lots of eggs, as opposed to the usual one monthly egg.
- About 10–12 days later she will take a 'trigger' drug to mature the eggs.
- Exactly 36 hours later – and this is timed pretty precisely to be early morning at the clinic – the 'egg collection' day arrives, the key day when her eggs are removed under general anaesthesia while you provide a sperm sample. (Odd how comfortable I am writing words like 'provide a sperm sample' when it actually means 'crack one out into a cup'.)

As I've emphasised many times, egg collection day is *the* key day for you, so make sure you find out exactly what happens on that day. Our first attempt failed because I didn't have that information.

If you lob in all that time preparing to do IVF, plus the difficult month listed above – with her taking powerful drugs to stimulate loads of eggs – if you are the weak link on the day, I can promise you that it's not the greatest recipe for a calm and harmonious relationship afterwards.

And just so you also know, events in the period after egg collection go as follows:

1. Eggs and sperm are mixed together.

2. The following day, hopefully some eggs will have been fertilised, creating embryos, and the clinic will phone you to tell you (or, more likely, her) how many there.

3. There will then be several days of speculative decisions by the clinic as they will want to put back the best (= healthiest-looking) embryo.

4. They will routinely check the embryos again three days after egg collection day – there will almost certainly be fewer due to survival of the fittest and all that Darwinism.

5. Ideally, they will wait until five days after the egg collection before they implant an embryo back into her womb, but if there are only a couple of strong-looking embryos after three days they will do it then.

6. 'Implant an embryo' sounds like a grand procedure but it's bizarrely pretty crude. You both go to the clinic, she sticks her legs in stirrups and the healthiest embryo is popped back inside her using a really long syringe in a process that lasts only about 30 minutes. No, really. That's pretty much it. You then go home realising that you have been sitting on a chair watching the conception of your child take place a few feet away.

Of the three times we did IVF, the pattern was:

- **First attempt** – NHS-funded
- **Second attempt** – self-funded

- **Third attempt** – NHS-funded (because, fortuitously, we moved house into a new district authority and discovered we could get another round of IVF paid for by the NHS. As I say, this was fortuitous and not deliberate... though had we known this beforehand I'm sure we would have moved house sooner).

The difference between NHS and private clinics

There's a lot of cross-over actually, as a lot of NHS hospitals do private work and vice versa.

The only real difference, though, was an incredibly important one: the standard of coffee.

That was as follows:

- NHS: first attempt, poor-quality, overpriced instant coffee from a machine.

- Private clinic: excellent-quality 'capsule' coffee from a machine at no cost and really quite delicious.

- NHS: third attempt, different clinic, good-quality, free instant coffee from a machine in a proper cup with saucer.

The joy of the fertility waiting area

Otherwise, the first thing to enjoy is the unique atmosphere of the fertility clinic waiting area. Like the silent fun you have in doctors' surgeries, you will inevitably check out the other customers/patients, speculating on the quality of their eggs and sperm.

The men would generally look fat, out of shape and old – obvious candidates for fertility treatment who you could barely imagine ever having the stamina or focus to engineer a single erection. And this, of course, is exactly how I looked to them.

What happened to us

The nice lady doctor

At our first ever consultation, on IVF attempt number one, we had a nice, neat and petite, quietly spoken young specialist who looked about 15 and gave off an air of clinical efficiency. Exactly the qualities you look for in someone to make a baby for you.

She took a piece of A4 paper, drew a pretty rough vagina (as it were, see page 83) and, in a barely audible but clinically efficient voice, explained the basic process of sexual reproduction. (This was an oddly relaxing experience, as I realised it was the first time someone had explained what happens inside our bits since I sat giggling about the whole thing with Julian Ives as a mid-1980s' schoolboy.)

She then went through the process I've outlined above, but in slightly more detailed and scientific terms.

The casino of life

The oddest thing at the time was that, at every point in the explanation, the nice lady doctor would give us the odds of IVF actually working, so in the end the piece of A4 was a biro drawing of a vagina surrounded by numbers and percentages.

We supposed this was necessary on two counts: probably legally to make it clear that there are lots of variables and lots of potential for the process not to work and, consequently, to temper expectations.

But it does also repeatedly bring home the greater oddness and odds of IVF – that, if you don't have NHS funding, you are gambling a lot of money on odds you would laugh at in any other situation.

Other fertility treatment options

Depending on your test results – whether there's an obvious problem with her or your seed – the consultant may then outline the other 'lesser' fertility treatment options.

You don't really need to know this stuff at the moment, it's just more acronyms, but if you do want to it's in the 'Her' section of this chapter.

YOU WILL BE IGNORED

As I've mentioned many times already, this consultation will be ALL ABOUT HER and not you. In the clinic's eyes, she is the one taking all the drugs and growing all the eggs, not you, so she is the focus of all the attention.

I was generally barely addressed. So get used to this – even though I can assure you it annoyed the hell out of me every single time.

I think it was just the assumption that as a man I wasn't equipped with the necessary emotional tools and requisite sensitivity to cope with the process. The problem with that is that it makes you feel like a spare part, an unnecessary intrusion, and also meant that, the first time we did IVF, I really wasn't as involved as I should've been, or that interested, because I was made to feel that I didn't need to be.

This book has been written as a His AND Hers survival guide with good reason. You both have to go through all this and the more you talk about it, share the stresses equally and try to support each other, the easier the process is. Hopefully, one day all fertility clinics will realise this and recognise that men aren't just a set of portable bollocks there to keep the other seat in their office warm.

An introduction to drugs

The specialist will also go through the list of drugs your partner will have to take and how to administer them. The first time you hear all this it will seem absurdly complicated. And that's because it is.

But remember that all kinds of idiots do IVF and if they can do it (and if we managed it), you can too.

How to survive this stage

* FIND OUT EXACTLY WHAT HAPPENS ON EGG COLLECTION DAY. Can't emphasise it enough.

* Ask to freeze a sperm sample in advance – and find out the extra cost of this. It will be an extra cost, of course (usually around £300), but is absolutely worth it to ease the psychological pressure on you on that crucial egg collection day.

* They will probably want another sperm sample anyway – clinics tend to want as recent a sample as possible – just to make sure all things are working correctly. They will also suggest (or even demand) that you do this at the clinic. This is a good idea to get a feel for the place and the surroundings and exactly what it's like in their wank booths. Chapter 7 will hopefully highlight the true horror of not being prepared.

* Don't worry about being ignored by the consultant. The process is about 90 per cent her, ultimately, so just try to be supportive and objective. It's not always easy, but try to remember why you're doing all this and resist punching them.

The consultant says...

It's important to leave that first consultation with a real understanding of the options available to you, the success rate of each of them and what they actually involve for you.

Do not come away from that first consultation regretting not asking something. Although, if you haven't asked a question you wanted to, make sure you have the means to get back to that consultant somehow to ask it.

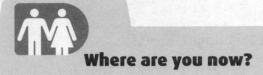

Where are you now?

You have had all your tests and got the results

*

You have been to the clinic, met a nurse and filled out
all the consent forms

*

You have met the consultant who will oversee your treatment

*

You (vaguely) understand the stages of IVF

*

You know what you will need to do at those various stages

*

Now a bit of info on the drugs she has to take and
what they do...

6

The drugs

HER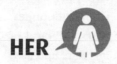

The drugs

Everyone talks about the drugs with IVF – the dreaded hormone drugs that send women mad and the terrible bruises from injections etc., etc.

But actually I didn't find them all that bad. It was certainly nowhere near as gruelling as the emotional stress.

It helps to know what they are all doing to your body, though, as there is a physical progression going on. As you move from one drug to the next it's quite satisfying to tick them off and feel like you're getting somewhere.

This section explains what they do, what they cost and the best places to get them.

What actually happens

This is a stage-by-stage guide of what the most common IVF drugs actually do.

1. Regulate your cycle

First, you may have to go on the Pill – this is just to get your cycle really regular so that they can schedule in when exactly you will be starting

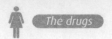

treatment and therefore doing the main procedures. I had always hated the Pill and never got on with it, but luckily I only had to do this in our first cycle of IVF as it was just part of that clinic's protocol. Not everywhere will insist on this.

2. Switch off ovulation

Next you need to 'down-regulate', which always reminds me of the Warren G song but in practice is far less glamorous.

This basically means they need to shut down your normal hormones and stop the natural process of ovulation. You do this by either sniffing or injecting a drug that basically suppresses your natural hormones. I used Suprecur (a brand of buserelin) twice and Synarel (a brand of nafarelin) another time. Other drugs you may use include Suprefact, another brand of buserelin, Lupron, a brand of leuprolide, or Cetrotide, a brand of cetrorelix.

I didn't find these drugs too bad. They made me feel a little bit drowsy occasionally but really didn't affect me too much. If you're injecting, it's usually once a day; if you're sniffing, it could either be twice or three times a day. I had to set an alarm on my phone to remind me to do this and once had to do my 'sniff' in the street, which must have looked pretty dodgy.

After about two weeks of 'down-regging' (that's what they'll call it on online forums) you go and get scanned (one of those vaginal probes again) and if your ovaries look 'quiet' then you're ready to start the most important phase: stimulating, or 'stimming'.

3. Stimulate ovulation

This involves injecting a drug that mirrors your natural hormones and which will produce and grow follicles that will hopefully contain eggs. I used Menopur (other drugs include Gonal-F, Follistim AQ, Merional).

It's the stimming drugs that are key to the process and give most women all the horrible side effects. Women complain of feeling mad and out of control with raging PMT-like hormones.

I didn't experience this at all. In fact, I felt slightly better when I was in the stimming phase as the drugs give you a boost of estrogen, which made me feel a bit more positive. Once you're in this stage it also means the end is in sight; your follicles are starting to develop and things are really happening in there.

Progress checks

All the time that you are stimming you'll have progress scans (yup, it's those lovely vaginal probes again) to see how your follicles are growing and developing.

The idea is that there are lots that all develop at the same pace and size so that you have a maximum crop at harvest time. Yes, the doctors really do talk about 'harvesting' your eggs like you're some kind of battery chicken.

4. Mature the eggs

After 10–12 days or so (this can vary quite a bit from person to person) of stimulating drugs your follicles will have reached the optimum size that the doctors are looking for – usually 18–20 mm diameter. Once they've got the majority of follicles at approximately that size (some will be bigger and some smaller) they will give you a 'trigger' drug of something called human chorionic gonadotropin, which does the job of maturing the eggs.

When we did IVF there were two different brands available, Pregnyl and Ovitrelle, and I had both over my three cycles. They essentially do the same job, which is to tell the eggs inside the follicles to mature and get them ready to pop out.

Timing is everything

The timing of this trigger drug is very important, as you need to take it exactly 36 hours before your egg collection procedure.

If you take it too early your eggs may be over mature or, worse, may start popping out (ovulating) before the surgeon has had the chance to remove them.

If you take it too late, the eggs may not be mature enough so you will have too many immature eggs, which don't make for good-quality

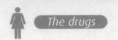

embryos. The consultants will tell you exactly when to take it and you must follow those instructions and not forget. There is no room for error here – your eggs won't wait and you want them to be just right when they are plucked from you.

5. Thicken the lining

As your natural hormones have been switched off you're now going to need a hefty dose of artificial progesterone to support your potential embryo. I was on Cyclogest suppositories but alternatives are Crinone gel or Gestone by injection.

What it does

Progesterone thickens your womb lining and creates a nice, healthy, spongy environment for your embryo to implant. It sounds quite nice, doesn't it? Not only is it usually taken as a suppository (up whichever end you prefer), but for me progesterone was the worst of all the IVF drugs.

Side effects

Progesterone made me feel the most PMT-like symptoms and made me feel quite low.

Unfortunately, this coincides with what many consider the worst part of IVF – the two-week wait (more about that in Chapter 10). Essentially, you're on a come-down now, and as well as a tortuous wait to see if it's worked, you have to stay on the evil progesterone that entire time and, if it has worked, for another 6–12 weeks afterwards.

Common IVF drugs and their side effects

Name	How it is taken	Effect	What it is for	Possible side effects
Follicle-stimulating hormone (FSH), Gonal-F, and Puregon Luteinising hormone (LH), such as Menogon, Menopur and Merional	Injections (one each day). When eggs are mature, you are given an injection of human chorionic gonadotropin (hCG) hormone to trigger release of an egg or eggs.	Stimulates the ovaries to produce eggs.	To stimulate ovulation before treatment cycles.	Over-stimulation of the ovaries (OHSS); risk of multiple pregnancy when used for ovulation induction, allergic reactions and skin reactions.
Nafarelin, buserelin and goserelin (also known as: gonadotropin-releasing hormone [GnRH] analogues or pituitary agonists)	Nasal spray, several times daily, or as daily injections or monthly 'depo' (injected under the skin) before, or at the same time as, fertility drugs.	Block natural release of hormones that regulate the natural monthly cycle. Produce low levels of FSH, LH and estradiol.	To stop the natural menstrual cycle.	Hot flushes, night sweats, headaches, vaginal dryness, mood swings, changes in breast size, breakouts of spots, acne and sore muscles.
Cetrotide and Orgalutran – GnRH antagonists	Daily injection under the skin. Given at the same time as FSH injections.	Unlike the pituitary agonists above, these drugs offer the alternative of blocking the release of FSH and are administered while the ovaries are stimulated to produce eggs in an IVF treatment cycle.	To stop ovulation until eggs are ready to be collected as part of the IVF cycle.	Nausea, headache, injection site reactions, dizziness and malaise.
Progesterone (including Cyclogest, Gestone, Crinone or Progynova)	Either after the injection of the pregnancy hormone, hCG, or on the day embryos are returned to the uterus, as a vaginal suppository, a pill, gel or by injection into the buttock.	May help to maintain pregnancy after IVF or IUI.	To thicken the lining of the uterus in preparation for nurturing a possible embryo.	Nausea, vomiting, swollen breasts.
Bromocriptine and cabergoline	Tablets.	Reduces high levels of prolactin hormone.	High prolactin can interfere with production of and the effect of FSH. Has a place even in IVF if prolactin level is high.	Nausea, headache, constipation, dry mouth, skin reactions, hair loss, lowering of the voice.

(Do be aware that this table is obviously not a substitute for proper medical advice and you should always speak to your consultant before taking any drugs and read all the available information on them and their side effects.)

Source: http://www.hfea.gov.uk/common-fertility-drugs.html

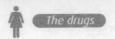

What happened to us

The idea of taking these fertility drugs can be quite daunting.

You know they are huge doses of hormones and you know that hormones generally affect your mood and behaviour so it can be quite worrying for you and your partner. You don't know how you're going to react and that's a bit scary.

My first ever sniff of the nasal spray felt like a landmark moment and I spent the next few hours trying to analyse my feelings to see if I had gone all weird. In the end I was lucky – throughout the entire drug stage I felt a bit low but I didn't feel mad.

I have heard others say differently though, so I think it's just best that you prepare yourself to feel really unsettled during this drug-fuelled period. Know that you will not be yourself but that every drug is helping you create your baby.

My hypnotherapist made me imagine the drugs as a 'golden liquid' magically nourishing my eggs. I guess it certainly helps to think of the drugs in a positive light anyway. Don't fear them and remember to do the opposite of that famous 1980s' anti-drugs campaign and 'Just Say Yes' instead.

Mixing your drugs

One thing I always wanted to have Richard around to help with was the mixing up of the drugs, because this is complicated. I had imagined the drugs would all come ready prepared, in some sort of injectable pen system that you just plonked into your skin.

In fact, increasingly you'll find that they now do and you might just have one readily prepared needle with a dose for each day. If so, this will save a huge amount of hassle because in each of our three IVF attempts we had to mix up the drugs ourselves.

Now, we are two fairly intelligent people with A-levels and degrees but still we found this responsibility a little overwhelming.

We were on a high dose of 450 units of Menopur (just one brand of the stimulating drugs you can be prescribed), which meant we had to mix up four phials of the drug with one phial of water.

This meant drawing up the needle with water and injecting it into the little phial of powdered drug four times, all the time trying to make sure you got all the drug and water mix-up (an expensive thing to waste) and had minimised the amount of air bubbles in your syringe.

As a perfectionist, you can get quite caught up in the whole air-bubbles thing. I spent a good long time tip-tapping the syringe like I'd seen on *Trainspotting* and squirting a little bit into the air like a true pro. Actually, you'd need an air bubble the size of a bowling ball to cause you damage and that's only when you're injecting straight into a vein. In IVF you're injecting into fat, so you're pretty safe.

There are various techniques to make things less painful, like rubbing ice cubes on the area before or after injecting to numb it slightly, but I found just pinching the fat was enough. Afterwards you can reward yourself for your absolute bravery with a great big piece of chocolate, as it's very important to treat yourself throughout this rather nasty process.

Injecting yourself

These drugs are almost always given as self-administered injections. The nurse will teach you how to do them but the first time you do it will be strange and a bit scary. Some people prefer their husband to inject them but I was happy to do it myself and didn't find it too painful as long as I injected into a nice pinch of tummy or leg fat. My preferred area was my thighs and I alternated legs from day to day.

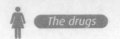

A bit about needles

When you open your box of IVF drugs you will be a little overwhelmed by the size and quantity of the needles. There are loads of them – and they are big. The needles look more appropriate for a horse than a human, especially a fragile, infertile and weary human.

But don't worry, look closer and you will see there are two sizes of needle:

- The big, frightening, yellow ones are for drawing up and mixing the drugs with the waters.

- The slimmer, pink needles are the ones that actually end up in your leg. And if you look at the tips of them you can see they are nice and small and seem a bit more manageable.

If you're still too freaked out to do it yourself, it's time to rope in your partner so you can think of something else and look the other way.

Scoring the drugs

Assuming you are paying for your treatment, the drugs are a substantial part of your IVF costs. Human gonadotropin doesn't come cheap, you know.

Your clinic will give you a drugs price list, which feels like a really unappetising menu and will allow you to keep things simple and buy them from their in-house pharmacy. However, most clinics will allow you to purchase your own drugs from their prescription.

This was a revelation to me and I got quite excited about the idea of shopping around. Did you know that ASDA sold IVF drugs? Yup, you can purchase a shot of estrogen with your fish fingers and chips (as long as you find a participating ASDA pharmacy).

There are also companies that deliver to you, which makes it all quite easy and discreet. We used a company called Healthcare at Home which couriered over our drugs at short notice as and when we needed them.

Obviously the cost of the drugs differs depending on your dose. If you're unlucky enough (as I was) to need quite a high dose of stimulating

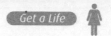
hormones to kick-start your eggs then you're looking at a pretty high drugs bill, as it's these drugs that are the most pricey.

Cost of drugs for a typical cycle

Just to give you a rough idea of the costs of the drugs, for our third cycle they were as follows:

Synarel x 2 £64.01 each = £128.02

Menopur 75 x 48 £11.60 each = £556.80

Pregnyl x 2 £4.05 each = £8.10

Cyclogest 15 x 3 £12.42 each = £49.68

Total: £742.60

(NOTE: This was, of course, my own personal prescription and your consultant will tailor the best drugs for your needs and situation)

A bit about eggs

One misconception I had before I did IVF was thinking that surely it was bad to take so many eggs out in one go? If you were taking out 12 eggs at a time, were you losing a year's worth of eggs and therefore reducing your lifetime's supply? Luckily, this is not the case at all.

Each month you have the potential for lots of eggs to grow and at the beginning of your cycle lots of follicles spring up. In the natural ovulation process they all grow and develop at different rates until, just before ovulation, the biggest follicle becomes the chosen egg to ovulate and all the others give up and retreat.

In IVF the aim is to keep all those potential eggs alive rather than just take out the one that's winning. So in a way IVF is about saving all the potential eggs and therefore just making the most of your monthly supply, rather than using up your yearly quota. Clever stuff.

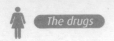

How to survive this stage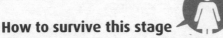

* Shop around, provided your clinic allows to you, as you may get the drugs cheaper elsewhere.

* Keep a tally of what you need to take and tick off each day as you do your injection so you can see you're making progress.

* Don't make any big decisions while you're taking the drugs – this is not the time to buy a new house, quit your job or, er, split up with your other half...

* If you are rowing more than usual with your partner, assume it's the drugs clouding your judgement. Park the argument for another time when you're drug-free.

* Even if you think you're fine, the drugs are quite heavy going on your body, so rest up, drink lots of water and be kind to yourself.

* Don't get disheartened by the scary needles or phials of powders, just take out what you need each day and before you know it your used sharps bin will be more full than your drugs bag.

* Numb or pinch the area you're injecting, and if you still can't bear it, ask your partner to do the deed.

* Reward yourself after each injection with a sweet treat – you deserve it.

* Set an alarm to remind you to sniff the down-regging drugs – if you're doing it three times a day you will forget.

* It's disgusting, but make sure you wear a panty liner when you're taking the progesterone – those oily capsules leak and will ruin your favourite pants.

HIM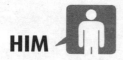

The drugs

For some reason, the only thing I'd really heard about IVF before we did it the first time was that the drugs she has to take have awful side effects.

'Like PMT multiplied by 90' is what most people I knew who'd done IVF helpfully told me. I was warned she'd be a bat-mental piece of irrational human wreckage, that she'd be teary, erratic and borderline insane.

In fact, for us anyway, this turned out to be rubbish.

But what you do need to know is how tricky the drugs are to administer and how bloody expensive they are.

And, contrary to that song, in this case the drugs do work.

I know, because, as a result of them, there's currently a baby growing inside my wife.

What actually happens?

The consultant you meet in Chapter 5 will explain what the drugs do and how they work.

You don't really need to know this bit but it will help you to understand what's actually happening. And anyway, if you show some interest while she's smacking herself with drugs every day, I promise it will prevent arguments.

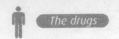

What the drugs do

(There's obviously more detail on this in the Her section of this chapter)

1. **Regulate cycle** – She might have to go on the Pill initially just to get her cycle regular. Rosie had to do this the first time we did IVF.

2. **Switch off ovulation** – The first IVF drug shuts down her normal hormones and stops the process of ovulation.

3. **Stimulate eggs** – After about two weeks she will then also take a drug to stimulate her ovaries to produce and grow follicles which will hopefully produce eggs.

4. **Mature eggs** – About 10–12 days later she takes a 'trigger' drug to mature the eggs.

5. Then it's egg collection day. May the force be with you and more power to your elbow, well, wrist.

6. After egg collection she'll be given progesterone – normally a naturally produced hormone but given now for several weeks to help the pregnancy. Or something...

What happened to us

The consultant will tell you the drugs regimen (they rather pompously call it a drugs 'protocol') that they use.

Their names are long and medical and meaningless. Some seemed to suit Rosie better than others. And they're really expensive. And that's about all you need to know.

The important bit is how they get into your partner's system and work their powdery magic.

Fun with powders

As I said above, the first drug (to shut down ovulation) that Rosie took was a 'sniffing' drug, and we didn't have the fun of injecting needles until a couple of weeks later when we took the egg-stimulation drug. And what fun that was...

That neat, petite consultant in Chapter 5 (the one who did the nice big biro drawing of a vagina surrounded by gambling odds) did explain – as your consultant will – how to administer the drugs, but you know you won't really be listening and so nothing quite prepares you for that first evening sitting in the kitchen with your partner's trousers down, ready to inject, as you try to work out quite what the fuck you are supposed to do with all these powders and all these needles.

Yes, there's eventually a bit of flicking the hypodermic needles to clear the air bubbles but, really, that's about as Sid 'n' Nancy as the whole thing gets.

Mixing up your gear

You see, rather naively, we assumed that the drug came ready mixed and ready to go, as increasingly that's how they're now issued to people.

Not so.

Instead, we had a pile of sterilised needles in two sizes. One looked normal-sized, the type you might see when you give a blood test at the GP's, the other was pretty huge, more like the type that would be used to put a buffalo to death.

Turned out the larger needle was used to 'mix up' the drugs, and the smaller one was intended for the actual injection.

Each nightly dose (I say nightly, as they suggested injecting early evening for some reason) came in four separate little glass phials, each containing a small quantity of powder. For each dose you had to break open a small phial of sterilised water, draw it up in the large needle, then squirt it into the first phial until the powder dissolved.

You then had to draw it out of the phial again with the large needle, squirt it into the next phial of powder and repeat the process – four times.

Now, neither Rosie nor myself consider ourselves to be total morons. There are many days of the week when I give an incredibly convincing portrayal of one, but I can spell and count and put on my own trousers and make a reasonable casserole. However, there are few things we have

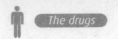
found quite so challenging as remembering the rules of this baby-making chemistry set. It still seems incredible that this stuff is just dished out to people to administer in their own homes because it's so precise, so measured, so fucking GCSE chemistry that it's remarkable that we're trusted with this stuff at all.

Because surely – by the nature of probabilities – this stuff will be used by anyone, including in the hands (or fists) of some totally clueless monkey sacks who are supposed to remember how to do this properly. I don't know if that is a factor to explain the relatively high failure rate of IVF but it might play a part.

How to inject

Assuming you have followed what you were told at the clinic, you should, some time later, end up with a small hypodermic with clear liquid in it, ready to inject into your partner.

Inexplicably (well, inexplicably to us), every time we did IVF the clinics suggested it was a good idea for the man (that's us) to do the injection, to take the pressure off the lady.

Oh yes.

Good idea.

And be assured that nothing says 'romance' quite like the two of you sitting in the kitchen with her trousers down and you hovering over her bare thigh (that's where they suggest injecting it – there or the bum – somewhere 'fatty', exactly the word a woman wants to hear in this context), trying to control what appears to be the early signs of Parkinson's while clutching a loaded hypodermic.

Not knowing any better, we took their advice that very first time Rosie had to take the drug – I actually held the needle and pushed it into her thigh and the sound of my loved one screaming the barely legible phrase 'STOP MOVING IT YOU MASSIVE FUCKING TWAT' somehow convinced us that me injecting the drug might not be such a 'good idea' and that Rosie would have preferred anyone to inject her rather than me.

112

Oddly, after a few goes, Rosie got rather proficient at it. She generally wanted me there to help mix the drugs and make sure we were doing it right but then she was happy (a relative term) to do it herself.

Get yourself an injector pen

Early on Rosie made use of an 'injector pen' thing that she was given by the consultant the first time we did IVF.

I'm not sure why, but on none of the other times we did IVF were we issued with one. However, if you can get one I'd recommend it.

It is a simple device but really useful as it takes a lot of the pain out of the injection. The needle is placed inside the spring-loaded device and you then place it where you want the injection, press a little button and it 'shoots' the drug in quickly and pretty painlessly. It avoids that little moment of trepidation, particularly if your loved one hates injections. Just a little note, as we discovered a little late, after Rosie had bought a box of needles, only one size fits inside the device so make sure you check them first.

Side effects

The most consistent thing you will hear if you ask people who've done IVF about their experience is the effect the drugs had on their partners.

I heard a lot of accounts of how they'd turn her into a turbulent bitch monster but, as I've said, for some reason Rosie had no side effects at all.

Maybe we – or perhaps it was just Rosie – were just lucky, but do be aware that your partner might react badly (mentally, more likely than physically), so even though we get ignored by much of the IVF process, this is another stage at which emotional support can be badly needed.

This stage, when she has to inject herself with drugs, is inherently strange. The key, I discovered, was to try to – politely – remind her why she was doing it and that it was finally the process of IVF under way.

It's also worth remembering that this stage only lasts for a few weeks, that the end is in sight and, despite what I keep saying about odds and chances and as utterly brain-crunchingly mental as it seems at the time, this is the chemistry set that really can end up creating an actual baby.

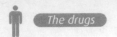

How to survive this stage

* Shop around for drugs – it can save you a lot of money.

* Make sure you know exactly what you're doing in terms of administering drugs, needle sizes, etc., before you leave the clinic. Get them to show you exactly what to do – it all alleviates the panic on that first time when you're both at home trying to work out the box of tricks.

* Be prepared for emotional effects on her – mood swings, irrational tantrums, rational tantrums, crying at a photo of a kitten in a hat. Yes, yes, I know you think you're used to it during that time of the month but, from friends who did experience all this, this is a whole heap worse.

* Be patient and supportive. Trust me, if you knew me, you'd know how hard it is to actually be either of those things. It's even hard for me to write those words. I'm a horrible, impatient, petty, vindictive wanker. Maybe you are too. But try to be nice during this phase. It makes life a lot easier and happier and a calm, positive mental state is massively important in IVF.

The consultant says...

Despite what you might hear, people tend to find that the drugs don't have a significant impact on them.

This is mostly because the effect of the drugs is to mimic your natural cycle.

The only one that tends to be an issue is the progesterone, because it can make you feel a bit premenstrual.

It's also important that people know the various options in terms of where they can buy the drugs to minimise cost. Remember, you don't have to buy the drugs from the clinic.

Where are you now?

You have met your consultant

*

You understand the stages of IVF

*

She has spent a month taking the necessary drugs

*

You may or may not have had a strange, turbulent past
few weeks

*

She has had the trigger drug and hopefully has lots of eggs

*

Now it is time for a trip back to the clinic to extract the eggs

*

This is the key day in the IVF process

7

Egg collection day

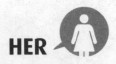 **HER**

Egg collection day

Egg collection day is THE DAY in IVF.

It's what you've been gearing up to for the last few weeks and months.

Everything you've been doing, all the tests, examinations, scans and drugs have all been about getting everything ready for this crucial day.

So it's essential, as far as you possibly can, to make sure that everything goes to plan.

It didn't for us. Twice.

What actually happens

You'll feel more than ready for egg collection day.

You'll have had numerous scans every other day leading up to it and you'll now feel like your ovaries are ready to pop.

You'll have had your final internal scan at your clinic and they will have decided if enough of your follicles are at a good size and they are therefore ready to 'trigger' you. This is the trigger drug that you take exactly 36 hours before your egg collection op. It matures and 'ripens' your eggs so that they are the optimum size and freshness ready for collection.

This may well be the nearest you will ever feel in your life to being a battery-farmed chicken.

Ideally, your scan will have shown up a good number of follicles that are reaching a good size. Follicles grow approximately 2 mm a day.

There will be some that raced ahead and some little ones that developed a little later, but the doctors are looking out for when the majority reach a similarly good size – around 18–20 mm. This is the perfect size to trigger and get them ready for egg collection. Basically, you don't want too many overdone or underdone, you want as many perfectly sized and perfectly ripe eggs as possible.

This is precision egg timing that makes even Delia look slack.

All about eggs

- The optimum follicle size before your trigger drug is 18–20 mm

- The ideal number of eggs plateaus at 15 – after that there is an increased risk of ovarian hyperstimulation

- The average number of eggs per age group at egg collection is as follows:

AGE	NUMBER OF EGGS
UNDER 35	12
35–37	10
38–39	8.5
40–42	7.7
43–44	6.5
45 AND ABOVE	5.2

Source: The Lister Clinic

- Egg collection is planned for 36 hours after trigger-drug injection – shortly before the woman's body might start to release the eggs.

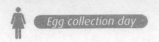

What happened to us

In all three cycles I had quite similar numbers leading up to taking the trigger drug.

I generally had about 15 follicles at a good size each time, which should have indicated a good crop of eggs on collection day.

During the first and third cycles I took a trigger drug called Pregnyl and did indeed retrieve a good healthy number of 'mature eggs'.

Too many eggs

On the second cycle I was given a different drug called Ovitrelle and this time I produced a whopping 27 eggs.

At first I was delighted, thinking I'd aced my IVF exams, and indeed the consultant came to see me in my drowsy state after the op and was clearly very pleased with the number and congratulated me in an excited whisper (so as not to upset the ladies in the neighbouring cubicles).

But I was soon to realise that this high number was a bit deceptive when it transpired that of those 27 only nine were actually mature. The others were either immature or weren't actually eggs at all. Who knows what they were.

All those mini eggs are no good for IVF and the sperm can't infiltrate them, so already my numbers were slashed by a third.

Ovarian hyperstimulation

What's more, there are risks involved with having so many eggs removed from your follicles – a rather horrible condition called OHSS (Ovarian hyperstimulation syndrome) which is when the empty follicles fill up with fluid and can cause sickness, pain and swelling that can be severe and spread so that you have to be hospitalised and have litres of fluid removed from your body. In severe cases it can even be fatal.

Some facts on OHSS

Mild OHSS symptoms are common in women having IVF:

- **About 33% of women develop mild OHSS**
- **About 5% of women develop moderate or severe OHSS**

The risk of OHSS is increased in women who:

- **Have polycystic ovaries**
- **Are under 30 years old**
- **Have had OHSS previously**

Most mild symptoms should usually resolve in a few days.

Source: www.rcog.org.uk/globalassets/documents/patients/patient-information-leaflets/
gynaecology/ovarian-hyperstimulation-syndrome.pdf

So, not only had I produced far too many eggs, I now had to take another drug called cabergoline to counteract the risk of severe swelling – a drug which can also lower blood pressure and cause dizziness, headaches, nausea and constipation.

Of course, in my panic at the time, I blamed the fact that I'd had a different trigger drug. But of course this was nonsense and it's worth pointing out that Ovitrelle is widely used as a trigger drug and clinics wouldn't use it if wasn't effective.

The actual procedure

Let me go back a bit to the procedure itself.

It's an invasive operation in which they insert a scanning probe into your ovaries and suck the eggs out through a very fine needle.

Then they pop them straight over to the lab, where the technicians take a good look under the microscope and count them up to see how well you've done. There is only a little bit of bleeding and cramping and your ovaries heal well over the next few days.

I had sedation the first time, which was fine as I felt completely knocked out (although I do remember lecturing the anaesthetist about camera lenses through my oxygen mask before I passed out).

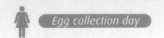

I came round pretty quickly afterwards but the downside of sedation was that the sore ovarian pain was there almost straight away because there was no anaesthetic easing things. On the second and third times I had a general anaesthetic, which I must say I preferred.

It really all depends on how you respond to a general anaesthetic.

I personally quite like the strange groggy feeling you have when you come round but I know it's not for everyone.

I remember having a very involved discussion about Spain with the Spanish recovery nurse the second time and about my puppy with the dog-owner nurse the third time. Poor them, I thought later, but they must be used to hearing loads of slurred, pointless rubbish.

Immediately afterwards

Once you're back in your room/ward again you are treated to a sandwich and made to drink lots of water and checked periodically for blood pressure, any pain, etc.

Meanwhile, your other half is being whisked off (bad choice of phrase) to perform his side of the bargain. They have the eggs, so next they need the sperm to get this show on the road. Of course, if you've read Richard's Chapter 7 you will know that this wasn't quite as straightforward for us.

Our disastrous first time

Let me tell you my side of that fateful day – our first cycle.

I came round from the op and whilst in my drowsy state I saw the nurse give Richard a huge metal incubator full of my eggs (surely they're not THAT heavy?) and off he went, full of purpose and good intent.

What was supposed to happen was that he would zip it over to the other side of town, drop off the eggs, fill his sample pot with lovely fresh semen and pop back to pick me up from the hospital, leaving the lab experts to make our babies.

But it didn't quite turn out like that.

We had already thought it could be a good idea for my parents to pick me up and take me to their home so that Richard could just meet me there rather than trek back across London. So, as soon as I was able, I travelled back with them so that I could chill out and recover while I waited for Richard to show up having done his duties.

Relaxing after the op

I settled into my parents' comfortable sofa and watched a bit of TV with them, with a nice cup of tea and a biscuit, feeling quite pleased with myself.

I'd been through all the hoops and made it to egg collection with, as far as I knew, a good result (they didn't tell me how many eggs they had collected but said it was all fine) and I felt that I'd done my part and it was now just left to the doctors to do their thing.

What could possibly go wrong now?

The *Nutcracker* ballet happened to be on so we decided that would be a nice comforting thing to watch. But by the time the Mouse King came on, I started to get a slightly bad feeling. I hadn't heard anything from Richard and it had now been a couple of hours. I had decided not to keep hassling him with texts but eventually I caved in and sent a no-pressure 'hi, how's it going? I'm all fine' sort-of text.

To which I got no reply. For an hour.

By this time we were on the final act and the Sugar Plum Fairy was in full prance. I sent another couple of texts but still nothing.

The knots in my stomach were getting stronger and, having now called and got no answer, the bad feeling was escalating, but I couldn't have imagined what the reason for his silence was.

Three hours later (now on to the 6 p.m. news) and I knew something was seriously wrong.

The phone call

My parents were trying to distract me with food and reassurances but I knew when I finally got a phone call that I was going to get bad news.

It was the nice nurse from the clinic.

She asked if I'd spoken to Richard.

'No...?'

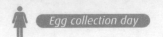

'I'm so sorry, but he hasn't been able to produce his sample and he's quite upset, he's asked us to phone you. He's going to try one last time but if not then we're going to have to close for the day and the only option is to produce a sample in the morning.'

My response

'Fuck fuck FUCKING FUCK.'

I think that was the first time I've ever sworn in front of my parents.

I started to experience quite a lot of heart palpitations and sweating. I tried to sound calm and think of some good questions for the nurse while I had her on the phone.

'What does it mean? Will my eggs survive the night? What are our chances now?'

Meanwhile, my mum, gathering what had happened was frantically mouthing at me, 'Can they freeze your eggs?!'

The nurse answered me as best she could and then told me I'd done really well and got 13 eggs – a very good number.

Great.

I'd produced a perfect crop of eggs and they were all going to sit there and rot, without a sperm in sight.

What a waste of all that time and physical upheaval, not to mention my shattered hopes and dreams. Crushed in one moment by the very person who wanted this to work as much as I did.

Richard.

Oh God. I could only imagine the state he was in. Not even able to phone and tell me. He must be devastated and anxious and stressed out of his mind. I knew this was a big, important moment in our relationship and how I reacted now was key.

How I tried to deal with disaster

I wasn't even really angry with him, just so upset that things had gone so wrong. I rang him and managed to calm him down a little and reassure him that everything would still be okay.

I didn't really believe that it would be but there was no point upsetting him further. I wasn't the one standing in the middle of London, in tears, clasping a heavy (now empty) incubator faced with the prospect of failure and having to do it all again tomorrow.

I decided to stay over at my parents' house so that Richard would not have the stress of me being there in the morning. He had to 'produce his sample', then be at the clinic when it opened early in the morning, which meant he would have to get up at some unfeasibly early hour to attempt to do his thing again. Awful. So instead we slept in different beds, in different houses, both going through our own version of hell.

I had a completely sleepless night, with most of it spent Googling for any examples of this happening and anyone having success with one-day-old eggs. I must have read some of the most obscure studies and papers buried away on the internet and none really offered that much solace.

The nurse had spoken of a technique called 'rescue ICSI' which she said the lab might try tomorrow.

They do it when conventional IVF fails, i.e. when no sperm fertilise the eggs overnight and so the next day they use ICSI to inject a sperm directly into an egg.

The numbers of fertilisation success with this were small, though; the stats fell down when it came to there being a 'live baby' at the end of it.

The morning after

The next morning I was hugely relieved and delighted when I got a text from Richard saying he was on a train, sandwiched between rush-hour commuters, with his sample firmly ensconced in a sock. (Presumably it was in a sealed container in a sock rather than just loose, but anyway...)

Thank God.

I was so pleased, not just because it meant our IVF journey was not over yet and we had some hope back again but because at least this was a more palatable outcome for Richard – he wouldn't feel like a complete failure now and he had managed to overcome the mental block by himself in the comfort of his own home. How I WISH we had thought that would be the case when we first planned it all.

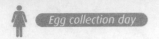

A thing called ICSI

The lab phoned and explained their plan was to try half the eggs with conventional IVF and the other half with ICSI and see what happened.

We panicked slightly about ICSI, because we knew almost nothing about it, but after some frantic internet searching we read some (largely unfounded) dodgy things about it.

Given the lack of other options, though, we went ahead with their advice and waited, relieved in the knowledge that now our job was over and we'd got there in the end. Even if nothing happened, at least we'd both finally managed to play our part in the process.

I'll talk through the fertilisation outcome in the next chapter.

Learning from mistakes

Needless to say, on our second and third cycles we came well prepared with a phial full of frozen sperm, produced at home and tested for quality well before egg collection day.

Both times, Richard attempted to produce a sample in the morning of egg collection day and both times he was successful. Just the knowledge that there was a frozen back up if needed meant the psychological block was alleviated and he was able to produce.

But he has never been able to produce a sample in a clinic – for testing or for actual IVF.

Get freezing

Now, Richard is a perfectly healthy, sexual being but he is also a sensitive soul and doesn't respond all that well to pressure. If your fella sounds similar, then be warned.

Think about all this well before you need to.

He might be fine, of course – and he'll certainly say that he is – so let him produce a test sample in clinic and if he finds that remotely difficult think about either producing a sample at home, or freezing some sperm – or preferably both.

It's too important a day and too big a deal to not have all your ducks in a row. If the clinic dares to dismiss your or your partner's concerns, make sure you speak up and use our example as a cautionary tale.

The man has a vital role to play and he needs to be absolutely 100 per cent sure that he can fulfil his side of the bargain – whatever that takes.

Once the drama of egg collection is over, you need to recover quickly and prepare yourself for the next few days, for this is when the fun really begins and you enter the rollercoaster week that is fertilisation watch.

How to survive this stage

* If your partner has any anxieties at all about his duty in 'the booth' then don't leave it to chance – freeze some sperm as a backup.

* Stock up on painkillers, sanitary pads and a hot-water bottle, it will feel like you are having a very bad period for a few hours after the op.

* Make sure you've timed your trigger drug correctly – it must be given exactly 36 hours before egg collection for the eggs to be at their prime during collection. Think PRECISION TIMING, channel your inner Delia.

* You'll need someone to drive you home after the anaesthetic and, depending on logistics, that may not be your partner.

* Book at least the rest of the day off work – I would suggest the next two days as well so you can fully recover.

* You will be bloated after the op so mentally prepare yourself from some insensitive 'congratulations' comments from people who don't know what's going on.

* Think positive – you've reached yet another milestone. You've fulfilled your side of the bargain and grown those eggs. Now it's up to the lab.

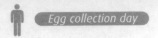

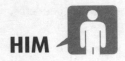

HIM

Egg collection day

I'm still not that comfortable talking about 'eggs'.

Sperm, I'm absolutely fine with. I know sperm, I have sperm, I know what it looks like and I know what it does. Sperm is sperm. Spunk. Man juice. But 'eggs' somehow seems wrong.

'Eggs' conjures up images of turtles struggling up moonlit beaches and boxes of free-range organic. They're things that lizards and birds and fish use to increase their number, not adult women. And surely not the one I'm married to.

Egg collection day sounds even more ridiculous, like a pre-Easter ritual for children, but that's what they call it.

I always referred to it just as The Day. Because that's what it is.

The Day, the most important day of the whole process, the day of days.

And if you read nothing else in this book, please, please read this chapter. Yes, it's long and explicit but believe me it could save you a whole bouncy castle of problems.

What actually happens

In rather crude terms, the process of egg collection is this.

1. For the last month your partner has been pumped full of hormones to make her produce more than her usual one egg a month. The optimum range is around 8–15 eggs (IVF success increases the more eggs you collect up to a peak of around 15), though, as any logical or kind-hearted embryologist will tell you, it only takes one good one to make a child.

2. The day before egg collection she will take a 'trigger' drug to make them all ripe and ready.

3. On egg collection day you both go to the clinic early in the morning and, with your wife either heavily sedated or under general anaesthesia, someone presumably experienced in these matters puts a long thing up her vagina, pierces the vaginal wall and sucks out each egg one by one and puts them somewhere where they won't go off.

4. It is then your turn to go into a cubicle and leave your deposit. This is then mixed with your lady's eggs to hopefully make some embryos.

But, as with everything in the IVF process, it is several miles from being this simple.

You are nothing but a dispenser of seed

As I've mentioned various times so far, one of the things I found most annoying about the whole IVF process was that I was just an unreliable seed dispenser.

Rosie and I still talk a lot about our disastrous first attempt at IVF and we're convinced that had we known then what we know now that first attempt would have been far more likely to work. Yeah, yeah, I know it's easy to say stuff like that, but we're certain. Carrying on down that hypothetical path we could now have a three-year-old child and this book probably wouldn't exist.

At every appointment before The Day I tried to find out what exactly it involved for me and was usually just fobbed off ('You don't need to worry – you've got the easy bit!') or just dismissed.

What happened to us

A little metal lunchbox

All I knew was that Rosie's eggs would be extracted and placed in an incubator which I was to take to the lab across town, hand to the nice people at the desk, do my dirty in a cubicle and then go home.

Now, it turns out that this isn't the usual procedure at all, it was simply because the hospital to which we were referred didn't have a lab of their own on site. They used one on the other side of town.

And this means carrying the incubator – which, I'm assured, is 'just like a little, metal lunchbox' – down the hill to the station and on a half-hour train journey.

The day of days

And so it was on the morning of 10 October 2011.

We arrived at the hospital and went straight to the assisted conception unit and the process began. I waited and, a couple of hours later, found myself sitting next to a bed, sunlight streaming through the window, as my wife awoke, dazed and glazed from the fog of heavy sedation. In a few hours she would feel the full discomfort of the procedure but at that point she was relaxed and fine.

A nurse soon arrived to check that Rosie was okay.

'Right, Mr Mackney, you need to get this off to the clinic,' the nurse said, pointing to a fridge on a trolley.

'Get what off, sorry?'

'The incubator,' she said.

Going back a week and describing the incubator to a nervous patient about to undergo IVF treatment for the first time, I think it's highly unlikely I would have used the words 'little metal lunchbox', more likely 'fucking heavy fridge with wires sticking out of it and an LED clock on the top'.

I made a squeak like Benjamin Braddock trying to book a hotel room in *The Graduate*, constantly thinking I must maintain my cheery frontage and do everything I could to keep Rosie calm.

'Right,' I said, thoroughly unconvincingly. 'I'll give you a call when I'm finished, Rosie. Probably just after lunch.'

The picnicking jihadist

The hospital was on a steep hill, about half a mile from the train station. And we didn't have a car. Or, it turned out, a trolley.

By the time I'd got to the station, my hand was in agony from the plastic handle of the massive fridge cutting into my palm and my right arm – the arm that on this day of days was really the key to us adding another member to our household – had been stretched several inches longer than it had been previously.

I stood on the station platform, fully expecting to look left and right and see several dozen other nervous men of a certain age avoiding each other's gaze while guarding their fridges and rubbing their sore hands.

What I didn't expect was the frightened faces of people as I got on the train.

Some moved a few noticeable inches away. All were eyeing me up, profiling me.

A few seconds later I got it...

My fridge was a metal cabinet. It had wires sticking out of it. On the top was a red LED timer. Now I understood the thought process going on behind their eyes:

'Oh shit. He's a terrorist who's come to blow us up... hang on, if he *is* a terrorist then he's a very middle-class one. And if he's not, he's really splashed out on a state-of-the-art picnic hamper'.

I remained silent of course, smiling politely, resisting the increasingly powerful urge to say 'It's okay, everyone, it's just a fridge containing my wife's eggs'.

The arrival

Twenty-five minutes later I arrived at a station on the other side of town. I dragged my fridge out on to the street and tried to follow the little blue dot on my phone map.

The clinic was on the other side of the station.

Of course it was.

And so I dragged my fridge up the road, round the corner to the other side of the station. But the clinic wasn't there. It was back the other way. Or maybe it was left there? Another 20 minutes later I found an office building which looked like it could have housed accountants or call-centre staff.

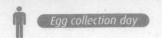

I dragged my fridge up to the first floor. I was exhausted and sweaty. I rang a bell next to a locked door with my unusually long right arm.

No answer.

Eventually a girl in a mauve surgical tunic opened the door and told me to come in. She looked about 15.

Some of them want to abuse you

I found myself in a tatty-looking waiting room.

The nervous men of a certain age that I was expecting to see at the station were here. Nervous, silent and avoiding each other's gaze.

The mauve teenager took the envelope attached to the side of the fridge and told me to sit down. Capital FM was playing Eurythmics through the waiting-room radio, slightly loud and occasionally losing frequency.

The room had the precise air of a sixth-form common room.

'Some of them want to use you, some of them want to get used by you. Some of them want to abuse you...'

To the left of the room was a door and a hatch. Over the next 15 minutes another mauve teenager periodically popped out and called out the name of one of my nervous comrades.

She then took the man aside and told him how many eggs there were in the incubator. Fairly personal and intimate information and within my earshot.

She told me that we had 13 eggs. A good number. The optimum number, she said.

But I also now knew that the nervous man next to me had four eggs. This kind of thing might be fine for competitive amphibians in a pond but I felt that I didn't want to know everyone else's fertility scores and that they shouldn't know mine.

Inside the booth of self-pollution

After a few more ova revelations I was called by one of the teenagers and taken down a hall.

The walls were covered with photos of babies. I assumed they had been created at the clinic by the chemistry of the mauve teenagers but maybe they were just photos of random babies Blu-tacked to the walls just to make this awkward band of seed-dispensers remember why they were here and so feel less grubby and pointless.

The teenager showed me to the last of a row of doors, told me to do my business in there, leave it in the tray behind the door and then someone would collect it.

She handed me a sterilised plastic pot. It looked slightly too small. Of course it did.

'And there are materials if you need them on the rack on the wall.'

I went in.

It was a small, dimly lit, narrow, windowless room with a hand basin at one end, a leather bench along one wall.

I saw the rack on the wall. Ah, there they were. The materials.

The materials are exactly as you'd imagine. I mean, EXACTLY.

Glossy jazz mags that have lost all their gloss and all their jazz. A rack of old, well-palmed crispy copies of such pre-internet staples as *Hustler* and *Razzle*.

The final box was ticked on the list of 'Things You Expect To Find In A Wank Booth'.

Visual aids

Luckily, I'd pre-loaded. Assuming there would be no decent internet connection, I had spent a rather tragic hour or so the day before piping pornography videos into my phone.

I was a little tired and my heart was beating a little fast, but I wanted to get this out the way so I could get out of there.

I looked at the time. 11.26 a.m. I could be home by lunchtime.

About four minutes into iPhone pornography time, I heard the door open and the same mauve teenager speak to me. I turned around while hastily trying to cover up my act of self-pollution (as if she didn't know what took place in this windowless booth).

The door was closed. There was no one there. She was talking to the man in the room next door.

Shitting hell. We weren't even soundproofed.

An audible hell

I became aware that a type of audible hell would shortly seep through the walls and into my head as I tried, using low humming and foot taps, to block out the unmistakeable sound of a man wanking next door.

But I could hear the man two doors down as well and I realised that I've never heard strangers wanking before. Or even – as if it makes any difference – people I know. All I could hear was a grunting, rustling choir of men bringing themselves off.

Focus. Focus. I just needed to get this over with.

'Just' get this over with?? 'Just'???

I was in a windowless booth in a baby-making factory. Images of *The Matrix* and *Brazil*, a production line of embryos to the backdrop of one of the most revolting soundtracks in human existence. It was a Monday lunchtime and I was stuck against my will in a paper-thin cupboard while men wanked all around me.

The man next door triumphed.

I heard him struggle with his cruelly undersized plastic receptacle. He washed his hands – how good of him – and heard the rustle of the bag as he placed his sealed deposit in the tray and exited the room.

Quick – a window of opportunity. In a few minutes another wanker (in the most genuine sense of the word) would be in there. But nothing. Nothing's happening.

Performance anxiety

I've never coped well under pressure. And pressure in the booth was mounting.

I decided to take a few minutes to detach myself from the situation. I sat on the leather bench.

What was the problem? There was no rush. I had a couple of hours if I needed them. There really was no rush. I just had to breathe deeply, think about other stuff, not worry and then get back to it when I was ready.

Besides, it's only wanking, the one thing over the last couple of decades at which I've been really successful. Nothing to worry about at all.

I heard the nurse again next door. Oh God. Another one. I tried to block it out and just relax.

'Just' relax.

A few minutes later I heard giggling outside my door. A couple of the teenage embryologists were sharing a little joke. The giggling faded down the corridor. I lay down on the bench and tried to conjure erotic imagery from my huge cerebral database and yet all I could see was my childless wife crying as our relationship slipped into the sand.

Nothing

Fast-forward three hours.

Yes.

Three hours.

It was now 2.32 p.m. and there was nothing happening in my booth.

Nothing, I mean, aside from a middle-aged man of my withered dimensions standing amidst the mushy, well-thumbed remains of his ego.

My tired, porny phone made a noise. A text from Rosie:

```
Just checking everything ok. Back home now. Bit tired
but all fine.
```

Oh hell, I thought. Don't reply. Don't do anything. She's worried. I know she's worried. Of course she's worried. A year we've waited for this. A year. With the last month pumping the veins in her legs with hormones.

One whole year.

And this was being paid for. We couldn't afford to do this privately.

This had to work. Come on.

But this didn't work.

There was nothing – absolutely nothing – going on downstairs.

Nothing. In fact, less than nothing. I was frantically thrashing at a tiny red flap of skin where my penis used to be. I felt desperately sorry for the poor thing. Three hours of violent shaking and strangulation. It should have been seized by social services and put into care.

A freak in a booth

It was now 3.32 p.m.

I had been in there for four hours, received three texts and a missed call from my wife, and could almost hear the last desperate breaths of each of her 13 eggs. My thoughts had now turned from running out of the building and leaping into the river to running away, getting on a plane or a boat, throwing my phone and my wallet into the sea and joining a distant monastery.

But I couldn't even leave the booth.

Leaving the booth meant walking down the corridor of Polaroid babies and having to explain what had happened to a teenage doctor in front of a room of seed dispensers.

I was now part-specimen, part-Victorian circus freak. I was now The Man Who Couldn't Wank and was absolutely trapped inside there on what was now one of my worst ever days on earth.

Blue salvation

Eventually – finally – there was a knock on the door. A tall doctor – who at least looks like an adult – peered round the door.

'Is everything okay, Mr Mackney?' he asked to an achey-limbed anaemic man by the washbasin who was as far from okay as he has ever been.

'No... I... just... I don't know...'

Oh bloody hell. My head was making all the noises of a man who was definitely about to cry. I tried to gulp down my emotions.

'It's honestly fine,' he said. This happens a...'

'It's not fucking fine,' I squeaked. 'I don't know what to do. This can't happen like this. It just can't.'

'Well, we could try giving you a Viagra tablet.'

And so I finally left my booth – feeling a lot like one of those Austrian children imprisoned in dungeons by their mad sex dads – and was led downstairs. The nice adult doctor handed me a blister pack containing one of those unmistakeable blue ovals that have been refreshing the parts that dirty thoughts can't reach for over 15 years.

'Just take it now and then get some fresh air, wander round the block and come back in about half an hour,' says my white-coated genital saviour.

'Okay, thanks.'

'And you can pay for it at the accounts desk on the way out.'

What? Was he kidding? Had he any idea what I'd been through? The certain end of my marriage and the live cremation of my masculinity. Surely – S-U-R-E-L-Y – he could have given me that one on the house?

Open-mouthed and sore-armed I approached a man at a desk with a card-reader and told him I'd been asked to pay for this tablet.

'Okay, that's £17.80'.

But my hand was now so crampy and numb I could barely type my PIN into the machine. I somehow fisted in four digits that appeared to work. He gave me a receipt. An actual receipt for an unborn child. What a nice souvenir. Perhaps they'd let me claim my £17.80 back if my son or daughter existed

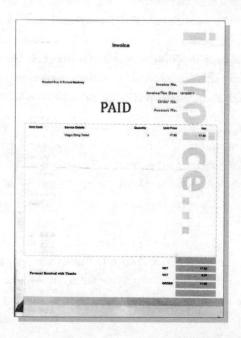

I realised I hadn't eaten or drunk anything since leaving home, so calm and carefree, about 96 hours ago. So I sat in a Pret-a-Manger and had a late lunch comprising a cheddar and pickle sandwich and an erectile dysfunction tablet. I wandered up the road and stared at that great, grey leveller, the Thames.

A booth with a view

About half an hour later, feeling slightly odder than I was anyway, I returned to the teenage call centre.

Another adolescent in mauve said they were moving me to another cubicle/room.

It was now about 4 p.m.

I assumed the other room needed to be wiped down for the next day's seed dispensers, though it'd take a scourer of rare efficiency to rid its walls of the stain of my self-destruction.

'This one has a view of the river,' says the teenager.

'Oh how lovely,' I didn't say. 'That should really get the blood moving into my cock.'

And so I was back in a booth. Another booth. Like the other one but in reverse. Above this one's leather bench was a window just as the baby nurse described, with a view overlooking the Thames.

Reverse flow

Clearing my thoughts of unnecessary contamination, I took out my iPhone and unleashed its sordid media.

After about 30 seconds or a minute, to my great surprise, I noticed that my poor, battered, scarlet genitalia was, if anything, even smaller and more scared than it was before my medicated Pret lunch.

Maybe the Viagra needed a few more minutes to take effect.

I sat on the leather bench and tried to think warm, gentle thoughts of lapping Greek tides and strolling along white sand in the long shadows of an evening in late August, our tanned bodies glowing in the orange light... and the look on my wife's face when I left the booth and told her that my penis didn't work.

And ten minutes later I gave it another go. Still nothing. If anything, even smaller still.

I looked in the mirror.

My face was bright red. My ears looked pink, fat and ready to burst. And my eyes were hurting on the inside and looked like one of the aliens in *Mars Attacks*.

My blood flow actually seemed to have been reversed.

Far from solving my masturbation issues that blue tablet appeared to have given me an erect face.

I used all the power of thought I could muster to re-direct my blood from my head to my lower abdomen.

Panicking, I lay on the floor and hoisted my legs up on to the chair, assuming, perhaps wrongly, that my blood was now anti-gravitational.

Still nothing.

Twenty minutes later there was a knock at the door. An Australian nurse with kind eyes told me that the clinic generally closed at around 5 p.m.

Oh great. It was like last orders: 'Can I have your spunk now, gentlemen please?'

Aware that my cause was unlikely to be helped by having people in my booth with me, hoovering around my feet and spraying Cif on the walls, I asked what options I had, staring the desperate stare of a man who would take, hands down, the Rose d'Or at the European Red-Faced Man Championships.

The final humiliation

I was told that the only alternative was to get some sperm to them by 8 a.m. the following morning and they could try then to fertilise the eggs, although they may have started disintegrating. The chances of fertilisation were greatly reduced but at this stage that was all I had.

I told her that I didn't know what to do about my wife. I couldn't phone her. If I told her about this it would destroy her. I pleaded with those kind eyes to phone Rosie for me and explain what had happened.

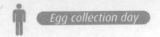

She said she would.

'Oh, the only other thing...' she said.

'Yes?'

'You do need to take that back to the hospital,' she said, pointing at the fridge.

Fucking shit-hole fuckers.

I had spent five hours reducing my ego and manhood to reddened mush. My right hand had almost gone into rigor mortis but I still had to save them the money for a courier. The final humiliation.

And so I went outside into the rush hour and stood on the pavement with my fridge and thought about the implications of this terrible day and the time and money we had lost and the deafening thump of the bodyclock and the crushed hopes of my wife and the unused baby clothes and our still empty spare room ... and I stared at the office workers and cried.

An evening of bloodless reflection

The evening was a daze.

A packet lasagne and a beer.

And silence.

Rosie decided to stay at her parents.

I eventually spoke to her and she was as understanding as any woman in her mid-thirties who's just had the fully funded hope of motherhood snatched away from her by a useless wanker in a booth.

I worked backwards; I needed to be at the clinic, fully seeded, by 8 a.m., which meant leaving home by 7 a.m.

That meant getting up and watching internet pornography at an hour when even the internet feels it's too early for filth.

Pornography for breakfast

And so there I was, in the kitchen. It was 5.30 a.m. and dark outside and my face was illuminated by the screen of an embarrassed MacBook as I clicked through page after page of various permutations of people pretending to enjoy sex.

And I began to realise how much I now hated pornography.

The silly plastic-titted fakery of it all.

The tired predictability.

The ugliness of watching strangers putting their nasties into each other. I hated pornography. I hated the noise it made.

And I hated breasts. And penises. And skin. And sweat. And I hated women. And sex. And men. In fact, all human beings. I hated people. I hated our grunting animalistic stupidity, our filth, our stench and our lies.

And as I thought of this vile species and what we'd done to this fine planet I clicked onto some Eastern European dating website and on to a video link.

There was a stocky young man hurriedly undressing a plump young lady in her bedroom. The image was clunky and badly lit. These people were real. Their hands were tearing at each other's clothes and he picked her up and pushed her on to a desk, both of them panting like hounds, hiking up her skirt as she ripped off her underpants.

And they both started rumping for England or Estonia or wherever this was and they were panting and thrusting and flapping around and having the time of their young lives and... hello? What was that? Well, where the hell have you been?

Suddenly there was movement.

There was actual movement.

The old fella was not dead after all. God. Bloody wow. This was just like being normal again.

I rushed into the bathroom, grabbed my undersized pot and, about 16 minutes later, I was sitting next to a window on a train to Waterloo and inside my jacket pocket, pressed against the warmth of my chest, were several million of me.

I texted Rosie and told her I was on my way.

She texted back about three point four seconds later with the unbridled relief of someone who had just been handed the very slightest hope of still being a mother. If I hadn't made that train and hadn't had something

in my pot to take to the clinic the gloom would have been impenetrable. But as I sat there by the silvery grey of that October morning, there was the faintest glimmer of hope.

I got to Waterloo and ran down the escalators to the Tube. It was rush hour, of course. I pushed my way to the ticket barrier, knocking the woman in front.

'Calm down,' she said angrily. 'It's not life or death.'

'Erm, it is actually.'

* * *

Brief hope

That early grey morning rush hour did revive hope.

Incredibly, despite my delay, three embryos were fertilised and two were put back for implantation (more on this in the next chapter), but a few weeks later, no matter how much Rosie wanted to believe – and even tried to convince me – that there was a tell-tale red line on the pregnancy testing stick, there was none.

I knew that The Day would now always be The Really Big Fucking Awful Day and the incident in the booth (I really hope they put up a plaque to mark the site where my personality dissolved) would mark egg collection day forever.

The world of frozen sperms

The second time we tried IVF, having explained to the consultant how our disastrous first attempt went, he said that that time delay and my long day in the booth would have pretty much doomed the chances of pregnancy.

But he added that the pressure of the day could be reduced hugely by just freezing a sperm sample in advance.

What? Freeze it? Hang on, where was that suggestion the first time round? Wasn't even mentioned.

The only hitch was that in the defrosting process there is about a 50 per cent fatality rate so there would be fewer semen to play with, as it were. The helpful specialist even said that, as some religions and races frown upon 'public' (i.e. in a booth at a clinic) masturbation, they routinely encourage freezing a sample.

So the second time round that's what I did – at a time of my choosing before egg collection day, I simply did my business at home, took it in and they popped it in the freezer, meaning that whatever nightmares occurred on The Day, they would always have a sample to use.

The clinic will routinely phone you about five days later to tell you the quality of your sperm and, if it's not great, you can simply do another one, and then as many more as you need.

Obviously there's an extra charge for this but, for that £300 (including one-year storage at the clinic), you avoid a whole heap of psychological damage, and the potential for wasting your time and money on one whole cycle.

Defrosting my offspring

Of course, the experience of The Day the first time round left its own scars.

On egg collection day the second time round, all was fine until it was time for me to do my duties at home. Suddenly memories of the booth were awoken.

Nothing was happening. Time was ticking and I began to relive the nightmare of the booth in my own home.

Yes. My own home. Oh please, no, I thought. Please don't ruin my only actual hobby.

They'd told me I'd need to phone by 11 a.m. if I was having problems.

At exactly 11 a.m. I phoned, shaky voiced and shaky armed, and apologised but this had happened before and I didn't think I would be able to provide fresh seed. No problem at all, they said, we'll just defrost the frozen sample.

And, freed from psychological pressure, just three minutes later all my parts started behaving normally and I was able to provide a fresh sample after all.

When I arrived at the clinic with my undersized, but fertile, pot (chest pocket as usual – they tell you to keep it as near to body temperature as possible) I explained the problems I'd had the first time to a nice embryologist who might have been called Emma.

She explained that problems in the booth were incredibly common. I told her that all the men I knew who had done IVF said they'd had no problems when providing a sample at their clinics.

'Yes, but men don't tend to tell truth about this to each other – it's not considered very 'manly'.'

FREEZE YOUR SEED

So good old effeminate me, a man seemingly immune to Pfizer's bluest and best, is trying to save you the pain when you do IVF.

And why didn't they tell us about the world of freezing the first time round?

But the above tale means it could happen to you, so don't let it.

We had to go through all the trauma and dissection of a failed first attempt at IVF, we believe, entirely unnecessarily. And we had to pay for a second round ourselves.

And that's not even taking into account the damage done to our relationship and my genitals. Not to mention the damage to my psyche by those five hours in the booth. I developed not just a fear of booths, but even a fear of leather benches, wash basins, the colour mauve, and magazine racks.

And I still go horribly clammy and experience slight shrinkage when I hear any early Eurythmics.

How to survive this stage

* Find out EXACTLY what the procedure is for egg collection day at the clinic you have chosen.

* Do not be fobbed off. And, if you are, perhaps ask the member of staff when they last had to masturbate under duress.

* Some clinics will encourage you do your first sperm sample on the premises – this will give you a chance to see (and hear) if you're likely to be able to do it.

* Make sure you do all this – it could be the difference between a failed first attempt at IVF and a successful one.

* In an emergency, think about perusing Eastern European dating sites. You never know who you might come across...

The consultant says...

Part of the problem with IVF is that we all like to feel in control but egg collection day is the stage when you have to put yourselves in the hands of the professionals.

The clinic should have given you an idea of the number of eggs you'll be expecting based on the AMH level and number of follicles on the scan.

It's also the first time when the man becomes part of the process. If there are any concerns about producing a sperm sample on the day, invariably having a frozen sample will minimise problems as all the pressure is off.

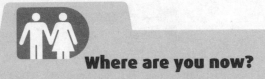

Where are you now?

She has finished taking all the IVF drugs

*

She has had the trigger drug to mature her eggs

*

She has been to the clinic to have the eggs extracted/collected

*

He has produced his deposit to mix with the eggs

*

You (hopefully) now have some eggs and sperm that are busy
getting to know each other

*

Now it is results time and a nerve-testing week of waiting
and decisions

8

Fertilisation results

HER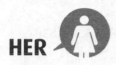

Fertilisation results

After the momentous day of egg collection comes nearly a whole week of stressful phone calls and risky decisions, during which you track the progress of your embryos and decide when to welcome them back into your womb.

This is where I think the term 'rollercoaster' really makes its presence known in the world of IVF.

It's a period of tension and anxiety and certainly the time that I felt the most stressed and out of control.

There is a fairly standard timeline of events that happens this week and, as always, it all revolves around numbers.

You have to hold your nerve and also trust in the advice you're getting from the consultants and the lab.

And cross your fingers. A LOT.

This is the most important game of chance you'll every play and bizarrely feels not unlike a very high-stakes round of *Deal or No Deal*.

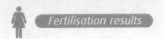

What actually happens

It's probably best to explain the process of this next stage using a timeline.

There's a lot of decision-making that is now done by the clinic to try to achieve the best possible outcome, but it always follows the timetable below.

Embryo terminology

Blastocyst – once the embryo has formed a fluid-filled cavity between the cells it becomes known as a blastocyst.

Morula – the stage before blastocyst at which the embryo contains about 10–30 cells. Most morulas are seen on Day 4 but some on Day 5, which are just taking a bit longer to become blastocysts.

Hatching blastocyst – as it expands, the blastocyst hatches out of its shell and begins to invade into the uterine lining to 'implant'.

Fragmentation – also called 'blebbing', is where portions of the embryo's cells have broken off and are now separate from the nucleated cells. It is normal to have some fragmentation, but embryos with more than 25 per cent fragmentation have a low implantation potential.

Arrested – meaning your embryo has stopped dividing and has died.

Inner cell mass – the clump of cells within your blastocyst that will become the fetus.

Trophectoderm – the outer ring of cells within your blastocyst that will go on to form the placenta.

Blastocoel – the fluid-filled cavity in the centre of your blastocyst.

Fertilisation timeline

Day 0

This is egg collection day.

It is also the day when they mix your eggs and sperm together, either via ICSI, IMSI or bog-standard IVF. This also counts as the day of conception and you will work back 14 days from this day to get your adjusted day of your last missed period, which is what will determine your due date if you get pregnant.

Day 1

In the morning you get a call from the lab.

This is more than a little bit scary. I have been known to shake while trying to write down the information I received on this day.

Some nice lab technician will do the formal hello, please confirm your date of birth and husband's name, etc., etc., and then they get on to the important news: how many of those eggs have fertilised overnight? You have to expect a drop off; it's hugely rare for all your eggs to have fertilised, but as IVF is such a numbers game, you want as many as possible to have turned into nice healthy fertilised eggs – which are now called embryos. On average, 65–70 per cent of mature eggs will fertilise.

Ideally, you want the sperm to have fertilised the eggs normally (producing two pronuclei – male and female) but there are a number of issues that can happen to disrupt this process.

Eggs can be immature (and therefore unable to be fertilised).

Sperm can fertilise the eggs abnormally (producing more than two or less than two pronuclei).

Sperm can fail to fertilise some (or, worst-case scenario, ALL) of the eggs, just because.

And sometimes what they thought were eggs are not eggs at all (which is mega weird and I never did find out what they were).

So now you are down either a little or significantly on your egg collection numbers and all your hopes are that the crop that is left will keep dividing.

Sometimes the embryologists in the lab will provisionally give you a time for your transfer on Day 3. They may advise you that if you don't hear from them on the morning of Day 3, you should come in as planned.

Day 2

Generally a day of rest. The technicians leave the embryos undisturbed to keep dividing. They should reach two to four cells on this day.

It's not particularly a restful day for you, though, although it is quite nice not waiting for a phone call. But you don't know whether you are going in the next day for transfer or two days later, so you have to plan for every eventuality anyway.

My main way of coping here was to think about healing my body from the op, ready to welcome the embryo/embryos back to me.

Day 3

Another terrifying early morning wait for a phone call. You're hoping for the embryos to be six or eight cells by this day. Any more or less could mean they are developing abnormally.

Then it's all down to numbers again. So bear with me for all the maths...

Basically (if this stuff is ever basic) they're trying to work out which are your best one or two embryos.

At this stage the embryos are also graded to give an indication of how good they are. Helpfully, quite a few hospitals have different grading systems, so make sure you find out whether a grade of one is good or bad...

The technicians look for evenly-shaped cells and also minimum fragmentation around the outside of the embryo – the more even and least fragmented the embryo the better grade it will get (never mind how uneven and fragmented you're feeling at this stage).

If that is clear by Day 3 and you have one or two obvious winners then they will probably suggest you put one or both of them back. The general feeling is that the embryos are better off in the womb IF you can tell which ones are the cream of the crop.

But if you are lucky enough to have more than two (often they like to see four or more) that are looking good then they may suggest you keep them in culture until Day 5, hoping that at least one will come out as the leading embryo and have turned into a great big juicy blastocyst (meaning it has now divided so many times it has too many cells to count) – which is generally what you want.

A blastocyst is a better bet for a successful pregnancy as it has proven itself to be hardy and has survived to a stage that is now ready to go straight on to implant in your uterus.

In our case the decisions were fairly straightforward. We had only two possible embryos to transfer on Day 3 in our first IVF cycle (an eight-cell and a six-cell) and Cycle 2 (an eight-cell and a four-cell), but we got lucky in Cycle 3 and were able to transfer our best-looking blastocyst on Day 5.

So, if you don't hear from the lab on Day 3, it usually means that the best embryos have selected themselves and you should go in for a transfer. But hopefully you will get the call saying many are still growing well and you should wait until Day 5.

Day 4

Assuming you're still in the game and haven't done a Day 3 transfer then Day 4 is another rest day for your embryos.

They are going through a stage called compacting, which means there is no point looking at them today and, already being treated like sleeping babies, the lab technicians think it's best not to disturb them unnecessarily.

All you can do is wait and see and pray (now that you've taken that gamble) that you'll be left with something to transfer on Day 5. And yes, even the staunchest atheists seem to start praying at this point. However, at least you don't have a phone call today so, again, it's a good idea to focus on resting up and healing your body and getting ready for the big day tomorrow.

Day 5

The lab calls with news of your embryos.

Fingers crossed at least one will have made it to blastocyst, although of course there is always a risk that all your remaining embryos will have given up after Day 3.

The only way to rationalise this devastating news is to know that if they didn't survive to Day 5 then there is no chance they would have turned into a successful pregnancy anyway, as every embryo has to go through the blastocyst stage to be able to implant.

In a blastocyst there is one-cell mass that becomes the baby and another that becomes the placenta. And, yes, you will see this on a magnified photo of your embryo.

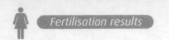

Blastocysts are not as pretty to look at as a nice, symmetrical eight-cell but they are already busy turning themselves into a baby, so you can forgive them this ugly duckling period.

Hopefully you will have one nice-looking blasto to transfer and you can go in for a Day 5 transfer knowing that your embryos have gone as far as they can in the lab.

Day 6

The lab generally keeps any remaining embryos in culture for one more day just to see what they do, as some can be a little late developing.

If you're in luck then some of your leftovers may also go on to become blastocysts. If they're of sufficient quality then the lab will give you the option of freezing them for any following cycles.

This is immensely reassuring as it serves as a sort of safety net in case this cycle ends in a negative result or a miscarriage – it means you can try again without going through all of the stimulating drugs (though there are still other drugs you must take to support a frozen embryo transfer or FET).

Or, of course, they can be kept for years until you are ready for a sibling. What is so brilliant about that is that they are frozen in time so in theory you might have more chance of success with your frozen embryo than with your own fresh eggs if you are significantly older when you try for number two.

However, as with all IVF dreams, nothing is certain and frozen embryos sometimes don't survive the thawing process. If only top-quality blastocysts are frozen then the survival on thawing should be around 90 per cent.

Unfortunately, frozen embryo transfers are slightly less successful statistically than fresh ones so it's best not to assume your back-up plan is guaranteed – in other words, don't put all your eggs in one basket (sorry).

More on the actual embryo transfer procedure in the next chapter.

What happened to us

Our numbers

Just to give you an idea of typical numbers, these were mine on each of our three IVF attempts:

- **First IVF attempt: 10 October 2011, age 35** – 13 eggs collected. Owing to the late sperm sample, they opted to do seven by IVF (two fertilised) and six by ICSI (one fertilised). An eight-cell and a six-cell transferred. Both good-quality on Day 3.

- **Second IVF attempt 27 March 2012, age 35 (just)** – 27 eggs, all done with IVF. Nine mature, which means 18 immature and only six fertilised. Transferred an eight-cell and a four-cell on Day 3.

- **Third IVF attempt 11 February 2013, age 36 (nearly 37)** – 15 eggs, two were 'not eggs' (what the hell were they then?) then there were four immature, leaving us with nine mature eggs, of which six fertilised normally. Got to Day 5 and transferred a blastocyst and one spare embryo to freeze.

How you will feel

As well as all the complicated maths, risky decision making and scary phone calls, you are also recovering from a fairly substantial operation.

I would highly recommend taking this week off work if you can – from your egg collection day to the transfer and a couple of days after that if you can. You may prefer to keep busy at work but, believe me, your mind will be full of fertilisation numbers, your body will be zonked and your heart will be with a Petri dish in a cold, dark lab somewhere.

Physically you'll be feeling the after-effects from egg collection and it's not just the usual general anaesthetic wooziness – your ovaries have really been through the mill.

Your stomach will be swollen and ironically you may look about four-months pregnant, so try not to slap anyone who accidentally shoots you a congratulatory grin.

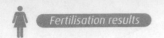

You may feel the pain in your ovaries now as they try to recover from being prodded and poked. I really did. The empty follicles fill up with fluid and this is when ohss (see the egg collection details in Chapter 7 for more on OHSS) can hit, particularly if you've had a lot of eggs removed.

Pamper yourself

I found it helpful to think that I should nurture and heal my body as much as possible so that the embryos were coming back into a nice calm environment.

So I had massages, did acupuncture, spoke to my hypnotherapy woman, had hot soothing baths and generally rested up and pampered myself as much as possible so that I could be in as good a shape as I could be for either the Day 3 or Day 5 transfer.

How to survive this stage

* Make sure you know roughly when the lab will call. Set your alarm and keep your phone switched on. You do not want to miss that call.

* Keep a pen and notepad handy as you will want to jot down the results so you can look at them over and over again and discuss them endlessly with your partner.

* Be ready for a Day 3 transfer, just in case. The lab may tell you to come in straight away so be up and dressed by the time they call.

* Take time off work if you can. Ideally that means the whole period between egg collection and a possible Day 5 transfer plus a day or two after so you can lie with your legs in the air (which of course won't have any effect on your embryos but will make you feel better).

* Book in something lovely to do on these days to help your body recover – a massage, an acupuncture session – whatever will help you to heal quickly.

* Don't be too disheartened if your numbers drop off quickly. As annoying as it is to hear, try to remember that you only need one good embryo to make a baby. It's a cliché but it's true.

* Visualise your growing embryos. My hypnotherapist told me they would need me to send them plenty of love and nurturing thoughts all the way over there in the lab.

* Drink! You've dedicated this last month or so to growing your perfect eggs and you may soon be growing an actual baby so this might be the last time you'll feel happy to drink alcohol. You deserve a big glass of wine.

* It's a weird time because your potential babies are existing outside of your body but they'll soon be back so get yourself ready mentally to receive them. You'll soon be pregnant until proven otherwise, so think positively.

* If the worst happens and you are left with nothing to transfer then take all the support and help you can. This is probably the hardest point to leave IVF and you will feel devastated at sliding all the way back to square one. Give yourself a break, recover, have fun and make a new plan.

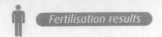

HIM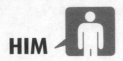

Fertilisation results

It's an odd feeling, knowing that in a room somewhere several miles away some people you've never even met are conceiving your child for you.

But the days that follow are, for her (and, therefore, for you too) the single most nerve-shredding phase of the IVF process.

It's basically results day, results of the exam of life and, like those recurring nightmares of school, the amount of revision you did or didn't do has absolutely no bearing whatsoever on your chances of success.

Nothing brings home the full stark reality of the lottery of life quite like the days after egg collection day.

What actually happens?

A load of mathematical probability kicks in straight after egg collection day, much of which you probably won't need to know (perhaps I'm a little slow, but it took me until our third attempt at IVF before I really understood the process).

Just in case you want to know the basics, here they are as a timeline.

Fertilisation timeline

The key days are the first day after egg collection day, then the third day and (possibly) the fifth day. You see? I told you it gets complicated.

Day 0

This is egg collection day. Her eggs have been mixed up with your sperm, either by normal IVF or via the other methods mentioned in Chapter 5 – ICSI or IMSI.

This, just for the record, is also counted as the day of conception. It's not quite perhaps the one you had in mind, the one that involved the randy, tanned version of you, a sun-baked foreign hideaway, a king-sized bed and an Olympic quantity of cheap booze.

Day 1

Singularly the worst day for her. It's essentially results day. Someone from the clinic will phone in the morning and tell you how many eggs have been fertilised, i.e. how many embryos you have. And you will hope to God that there are some.

Day 2

Consider it a day of rest. The lab leave the embryos to do what embryos do when left alone in a dish: the healthy ones will carry on dividing cells, the unhealthy ones will slow down and probably die. This obviously means that with each day there will be fewer embryos.

Day 3

The clinic checks the embryos again and give you/her another call. More cause for nerves to do what nerves do when faced with life-changing news. Ideally the clinic will wait another couple of days to Day 5. Day 5 is the optimum day as by this point a good embryo will have matured to an advanced state known as 'blastocyst'. You will hear that word a lot this week. I always thought it was a stupid term that sounded like an exploding zit. Anyway, blastocysts are good things; they are embryos that have a very good chance of turning into babies.

However – and this is where it all turns a bit fertility game show – if on Day 3 there are only a couple of good healthy embryos left, the clinic may prefer to implant them on this day as it is assumed embryos have a better chance of long-term survival in wombs rather than laboratory pots.

This means you need to be prepared to go back to the clinic on this day but you won't know until the actual morning if you have to or not. If there are more than two healthy looking embryos they may decide to wait until Day 5.

Day 4

Another day of rest as the clinic (and you) hope they've made the right decision to wait until Day 5.

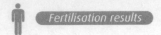

Day 5

Another phone call from the lab to hopefully say you have one of those blastocysts. If so, it's off to the clinic for the implanting – they call it 'embryo transfer' – which is explained in the next chapter.

What happened to us

All the above sounds like an orderly process, and mostly it is, but it ignores the thousands of variables that go with IVF and it doesn't take into account human emotions.

That first time we did IVF (described in ruthlessly foul detail in the previous chapter) we knew that hopes of creating a baby were rather thin. Rosie's eggs had sat in the lab, very much unfertilised, for 24 hours and my seed was nearly a day late.

A thing called 'ICSI'

Contrary to the above timeline, we were phoned about an hour after I delivered my tiny pot of sperm.

The technicians explained, in diplomatic terms, that the circumstances weren't really ideal (probably actually wanting to just say 'it took you over a day to successfully wank, you idiot') and to maximise chances of fertilisation they'd like to fertilise half of the four surviving eggs via IVF and half via something called 'ICSI'.

I've mentioned that acronym a few times but on that grey morning as I made my way home after one of the most bizarre and stressful 24 hours I'd ever had, I had no idea what ICSI was. Neither did Rosie. But we had to decide within an hour what to do and to give them a call back and let them know.

But all this was new to us.

We didn't really understand what IVF was, and just assumed they lobbed all the sperms and eggs together in a big dish and hoped the fastest and strongest made it through.

So with Rosie at home and me walking along the Thames we mutually trawled the internet trying to find out what ICSI was and whether there were any risks involved in doing it.

From what we could discover, it meant they wanted to isolate one good-looking, fast-swimming healthy sperm from the pack and inject it directly into one of Rosie's eggs. This would raise the chances of fertilisation, saving the poor little sod the battle to get through the egg wall (or egg shell?).

But there were risks according to some results thrown up by Google.

The technique was fairly new, I read as I strode along the river so there wasn't a lot of data and case studies to work from but... someone in the States had done research to show there was a slightly higher chance of hereditary issues with ICSI babies.

Shit.

'Issues.'

But what 'issues'?

Maybe this could all mean that we might be fertilising an egg and creating a baby just because we could.

This might not be a healthy baby. It might be a little slow, a dunce, a thicky, the one bullied in class for poor hygiene and bad spelling, the last to be chosen for the football team, and all because we wanted something to show for our horrible last few months.

I phoned a friend of mine who I knew had done IVF and remembered that she and her husband had used some other technique than usual IVF.

I explained the situation and that we had about 38 minutes left to decide the fate of our unborn child.

She had done ICSI, she told me, and had a lovely three-year-old daughter to show for it. The only ICSI issues she and her husband had heard about was the slight risk of a low sperm count if the father had a similar problem. Otherwise, nothing. The ICSI risks we'd read about were 'horse shit' and had been widely discredited. Go for it, she told me. So we did.

And so in about 51 pretty hideous minutes Rosie and I had decided the fate of our unborn, and had played conception roulette while simultaneously becoming amateur embryologists, gene splicers, experts in our field.

We would later learn, however, that we had been probably wasting our time anyway.

As I've said, the second time we did IVF the consultant suggested that given the time delay between sperm and egg finally meeting, the chances of a healthy embryo had been vastly reduced. But it gives an insight into the whirlwind of madness that can suddenly ensue. Huge decisions made at huge speed and then gambling on them.

The phone calls

One other thing you really need to know. Those phone calls – the day after egg collection day and subsequent calls – are, bereavement aside, some of the most difficult phone calls a woman will ever receive.

They are effectively telling her whether she should still have hope or whether she will have to remain childless until another attempt or forever. Not the easiest call to take.

I couldn't possibly comprehend what Rosie was going through. I tried, of course, but what comparison is there? That job you really want? The dream holiday or cash pile you might have won? Or maybe it was more like that call telling you whether your cancer is treatable or not. I have no idea. I just dreaded them because I knew what the wrong result would mean for her.

Rosie would barely sleep the night before and would be shaking when her phone rang. Luckily, in all our three attempts at IVF, the people who phoned from the different clinics were very well practised in the art of quiet reassurance, calm and professional tacticians highly accustomed to the anxieties of would-be mothers.

We were also lucky in that, even that disastrous first time, there were always embryos. Embryos that subsequently wouldn't survive at various stages, but at least they gave us some hope for a few more days or weeks.

I have no idea the hell that a woman must go through when she receives this phone call and the clinic tells her there were no eggs fertilised, but it's worth remembering that such a situation is unusual as the clinic will do all they can (using that ICSI technique if necessary) to make sure some sperms meet some eggs.

If embryos don't survive, remember it's for good reason. Nature is very clever at filtering out the healthy from the deficient.

It's child-making biology at its most stark and crude but if you get to Day 3 or Day 5, you will be heading for the next stage, where you actually get to watch your child's first appearance on telly.

And who said there was never anything interesting on TV?

How to survive this stage

* Easy to say, but try to prepare yourself (and her) for disappointment. If embryos don't survive it is for very good reason: they simply weren't healthy enough and they wouldn't have ever made healthy babies anyway.

* I know I keep saying it, but be as supportive as you possibly can be. This is a nightmare of a week for her. Men have no idea what all this actually feels like. We don't have the biological clock or that maternal urge. Keep her cheery and as positive as possible. Make dinner, watch funny films, pamper her. I promise you, I'm pretty crap at all that stuff too, but try. It helps.

* There is also a fair bit of physical repairing that begins now. Rosie was in quite a lot of pain after each egg collection day. Be aware that a surgeon has been probing around, sucking eggs out of her vaginal wall so it's, er, fairly understandable. Make sure she takes it easy, and try to get her to take a week off work at this stage. These are not phone calls you want to be receiving while in a busy office full of twats.

The consultant says...

Waiting for that results phone call, you will be on tenterhooks, but it's important that you're not too disheartened if the result isn't what you expected.

Remember, the aim of all of this is to get one or two nice embryos. Some women may only get two eggs but they could both be fantastic embryos, some women may get ten eggs but only end up with one nice embryo.

This is a key point but it's not the deciding day.

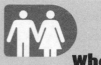

Where are you now?

You have survived egg collection day – singularly the most important day of the whole IVF process

*

You have survived the waiting and (hopefully) got a few healthy embryos

*

You are now nearly at the end of the process

*

Now it is time to implant one or two of the embryos into her womb

*

It is okay, it is nowhere near as painful or as complex as that sounds

9

Embryo transfer

HER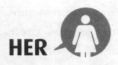

Embryo transfer

The is the final stage in the IVF process, at least medically.

After this you are essentially back to being a 'normal' person who has conceived naturally and has a fertilised egg on board waiting to develop into a potential human being. WOW!

You may feel sad that the medical profession can't take you any further on your journey, but they've done their bit, forcing your eggs and sperm together, and now they will check your lining is nice and thick and pop the embryos in.

Then they hand you back to Mother Nature and, I'm afraid, you just have to wait.

What actually happens

A positive thought

The main thing to remember at this stage is that you've got this far.

You've been through so many hoops to get here – the drugs, the scans, the injections, the invasive egg-collection procedure and sperm sample pressures, the lab results, fertilisation and then waiting for your embryos to develop.

You've been through so much, so many pitfalls and hurdles and you've aced them all. And now, finally, you're here.

You may have a Day 3 transfer or a Day 5 transfer (as discussed in the previous chapter) and you may be having one or two embryos put back in, but the procedure is the same.

Possible preparations

Hopefully you're feeling ready to receive your embryos and that your body is a bit recovered from the egg collection op.

Some people swear by having acupuncture just before and/or just after embryo transfer. This is because of a study that showed that acupuncture at those times made you more likely to have a positive pregnancy test result. However, this was just one study and as with all studies and statistics, it wasn't definitive and could be interpreted in a number of different ways.

It was compelling, especially to a desperate hormonal woman, and I deliberated over this one a lot.

I spoke to the acupuncturist who had helped me during IVF about it. We decided that actually the most important thing was that I was as relaxed as possible. For me, getting in the car and driving over to see her both before and after my transfer would not have been conducive to creating a relaxed atmosphere for my womb.

So instead I had acupuncture the day before and as soon afterwards as was convenient. My instinct was to go straight home after transfer and put my feet up. I would definitely say to follow your instincts on this one – if it will relax you to have acupuncture then do that, but otherwise be guided by what will make you feel most chilled out. We don't know much about the whys and hows of implantation but we can guess that those tiny embryos want a nice relaxed womb.

Ultimately, it's nice to try to approach this day with as much positivity as possible. From now on there will be less science involved and more blind hope, so you may as well get on board with the idea that a positive attitude and good vibes can only be a good thing.

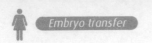

To single embryo transfer or not to single embryo transfer, that is the question...

If you are being called in for a Day 3 transfer, it is at this stage that you must decide whether to have one or two embryos put back (assuming you have two to choose from).

In the UK, the HFEA guidelines are that a maximum of two embryos can be transferred to women under the age of 40 and a maximum of three can be transferred in women aged 40 and over.

But they are very keen on elective single embryo transfer where possible, to reduce the risks associated with multiple births.

In general, the advice seems to be that you should transfer two embryos (if you have them) on Day 3 but should really only transfer one blastocyst (if you have one) on Day 5.

The reason for this is that the blastocyst has much more likelihood of going on to be a successful pregnancy, whereas there are more hoops for your embryo to go through at the Day 3 stage and so you might well assume that only one will make it to a blastocyst.

Ideally the medical profession deems it safer for you and your babies if you can have them one at a time rather than all in one go.

However, which IVF woman hasn't daydreamed about twins and a ready-made family in one go?

The procedure

The actual transfer procedure itself is quick and fairly painless.

You'll go into your clinic with your partner and then into a room with your consultant and perhaps a nurse as well. They'll talk to you about how nice-looking your embryo is (or are, if there are two) and discuss with you which one or two you are putting back.

You usually have to sign a consent form at this stage to confirm how many you are having transferred.

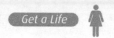

You'll probably be pretty obsessed with analysing what they think your chances are. After all, they've seen thousands of tiny embryos and surely must have an inkling which ones are going to make it into babies and which aren't.

However, IVF doctors are generally as non-committal as they can be. They can see the desperate hope in your eyes and will not want to lead you either way if they can help it. Hopefully you'll have a nice, positive consultant who will be encouraging about your embryos.

What you need to hear now is good news and feel good vibes. These aren't just embryonic cells to you, they are potential human beings, the children you've always dreamt of during the many years leading up to this point. You need to believe in them.

That's why the odd little comment – however well intended – can have huge psychological repercussions, as we experienced during one of our cycles.

Pregnancy rate for the number and stage of embryos transferred

	Elective single embryo transfer (eSET)		Double embryo transfer	
	Cleavage (Day 3)	Blastocyst (Day 5)	Cleavage (Day 3)	Blastocyst (Day 5)
18–34 years	33.5%	48.9%	36.8%	50.7%
35–37 years	28%	47.1%	33.8%	48.6%
38–39 years	22.4%	38.8%	27.3%	42.9%
40–42 years			18.6%	37.0%
43–44 years	13.5%	30.7%	9.4%	25.0%
45+ years				
All ages	30.3%	47.1%	30.9%	46.0%

Figures are aggregated owing to the small numbers involved.

Source: www.hfea.gov.uk/docs/HFEA_Fertility_Trends_and_Figures_2013.pdf

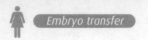

What happened to us

There I was lying back on the couch with my legs dangling awkwardly in stirrups when the consultant doing the transfer said, *en passant,* that she thought it was strange that all our embryos had started disintegrating so quickly (we'd gone pretty rapidly from nine to two) and had we considered doing DNA fragmentation testing on Richard's sperm?

What, what, what?

What did she say??

What is DNA fragmentation and how come we've never heard of it?

What does it mean?

What does the test involve?

What are the consequences if he does have it?

Oh, and by the way, thanks so much for casually dropping a great big shitty panic bomb into the conversation when I am just about to welcome our (now obviously crap) embryos back inside me.

Instead of thinking happy positive thoughts about nurturing our growing babies on the car journey on the way home I found myself scrabbling around the internet searching for the words 'sperm DNA frag tests' and reading some fairly discouraging statistics.

Hopefully this won't happen to you, but just be aware that careless comments are sometimes made – remember that the clinic staff are scientists doing a pretty important job – and try not to read too much into them.

Anyway, back on the couch, you lie back and get into a similar position as if you're having a smear – i.e., embarrassing and undignified.

But don't think about that, think about your tiny embryos coming back to you, where they belong and where you can nurture them into actual living beings.

When you and the consultant are ready there is usually some surreal activity where an embryologist suddenly appears (often from behind a hatch, like a baby drive-thru) and asks you both to confirm your names and dates of birth.

They have to go through rigorous checks to make sure there is no embryo/identity mix up for obvious reasons. Mistakes have happened (although very rarely) in the past so they have a number of checks in place.

Once you've identified yourself they hand your precious embryos on a long catheter to the consultant who very carefully slides them into your uterus and pops them safely on to your womb lining.

Sometimes they do this via ultrasound so you can actually see them going into place, but don't get too excited about this, as they just look like tiny dots and you can't really feel any connection with them at this point.

But, if you're a bit of a control freak (hello, me) it is nice to see them actually go in as it can all seem a bit surreal at this point.

Then the consultant very carefully removes the catheter and the embryologist checks it under the microscope to make sure none of them got stuck in there. Once everyone's happy you can finally put your legs back together and get up.

Embryos in and off you go

There are some schools of thought that believe you should lie there and rest for a bit, but the three clinics I went to were happy for me to just get up and get on with my day.

Even though you will feel like the embryos can fall out, and will develop a strange pregnancy waddle just in case, be assured that they can't.

Someone gave me the analogy of it being like putting a grain of salt into a peanut-butter sandwich, which, although fairly odd, did resonate with me that they were safely attached to my lining (I'm not sure if it is technically as sticky as peanut butter but it's a nice thought).

Your first photo

They usually give you a photo of your embryo/embryos as well, which we always found weird.

The first time we had the embryo transfer the printer didn't work so we didn't get a photo but the second and third times we got lovely little

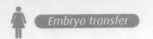

pictures with their own little frames. Yes, really.

It does make you feel a bit odd – where most people's first 'photo' of their baby is their 12-week ultrasound scan picture with identifiable limbs, head and nose, you have a picture of your 'baby' as a jumble of cells, like this:

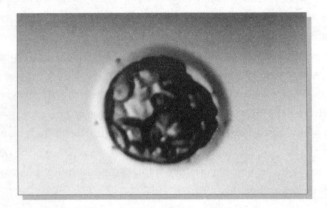

It's hard to identify with but by this stage in your fertility marathon you'll cling to any positives, no matter how bizarre.

Besides, you need something tangible to see you through the next couple of weeks of worry, so stick the photos on your fridge and look at them every day.

Afterwards

Now, it's up to you.

Apart from the progesterone suppositories (nice), you are now drug-free and you won't speak to your clinic for another ten days or so when you will phone up with your pregnancy test result.

For the next couple of weeks, sister, you're on your own.

You might feel elated, scared or even numb. The important thing is that you've reached this significant milestone and you are now a wonderful acronym: PUPO (Pregnant Until Proven Otherwise).

How to survive this stage

* Apparently your delicate little embryos aren't that keen on strong odours and your clinic might tell you not to wear perfume. However, it's increasingly rare that your clinic will ask you to do this.

* Take in some relaxing music on your phone so you can stay as Zen as possible, despite the fact that you're lying under bright lights, legs akimbo.

* Wear loose clothes that are easy to slip on and off. The last thing you'll want to be doing with your precious embryos on board is to squeeze yourself into ill-fitting trousers.

* Go straight home afterwards and lie on the sofa. You don't need total bed rest but at least put your feet up and relax for that afternoon.

* It would be unwise to cough or sneeze while the catheter is going in, so if you've got a cold, warn your clinic first.

* Get your partner to brush up on his stand-up (or sit-down) comedy routine. There was a small study that showed a greater implantation success rate when patients were visited by a clown during embryo transfer, suggesting that laughter really is the best medicine.

* Get a lift home, you will not want to be bumped into on public transport as you will be hyper-conscious of keeping your embryos in place.

* Watch some feel good films that raise your endorphins and help your embryos to settle in. For example, on my third IVF cycle I watched a delightfully unchallenging Jennifer Aniston film where she gave birth to a baby she named Molly – I like to think of that as a sign.

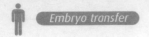

HIM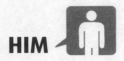

Embryo transfer

This is final stage of the medical bit of the process.

You go back to the clinic, they pop an embryo into your partner and you go home and wait.

It sounds simple and, actually, from experience, it is.

Oh, and they sometimes show the process on a TV screen. You actually watch them extend your family tree; the evolution will be televised.

What should happen

It always felt like this should be the day of clinical precision and scientific excellence.

A day of geneticists and specialised laboratory technicians, experts in their field, clad in sterile UV masks and hypoallergenic suits nervously whispering to each other as they carefully release the sealed lid of a vast metal chamber.

With a hiss, amid the cascades of dry ice, they extract a miniature vacuum canister, at the centre of which is a human embryo.

Aware that time is against them and that precision is everything, years of experience take over as they gradually but purposefully transfer this fragile mass of cells, the chosen one, from its clinical womb to the lining of its mother.

What actually happens

In reality, you go into a room, she pulls off her trousers and pants, lies on the bed and a man or woman – who you assume has some experience of this procedure – is handed a syringe and squirts its contents up inside her.

That's honestly pretty much it.

No teams of experts, no vacuum containers, no dry ice, no drama, not even a surgical mask.

I can only vaguely remember them putting on rubber gloves.

What happened to us

The call from the clinic will come on the morning of the third or fifth day after egg collection (see the previous chapter for an explanation of how that decision is made), and you'll have to go in as soon as you can.

The first time we did IVF, before receiving the call we knew that because of my delayed fertilisation hopes of the embryos actually becoming babies were fairly slim.

On the third day, clearly presuming that none may make it much further, the clinic called and suggested putting two embryos back that day.

Obviously, this being our first time, Rosie was nervous but knew she shouldn't be. This was, after all, the end of the whole process – at least medically.

Our baby, admittedly in pretty basic, multi-celled form, was being implanted into its mother's womb and nature would be left to take over. Finally we were at the stage reached by people who conceive without IVF, the key difference being that they usually don't know it's happened.

Rosie put loads of effort into trying to be relaxed and positive, to give the little thing a warm, friendly welcome.

She had read lots of material about a positive mental attitude having a subliminal effect on the embryo's chance of implanting, deciding it was a nice place to stay and then growing into a baby human. I agree with all that stuff, as naff as it can feel at the time, and did my best not to behave like my default self – a miserable old shitter.

She had also read that wearing any product with scent could interfere with the embryo as it was being transferred so I was told – well, ordered, actually – not to put on any deodorant.

She also told me that I'd have to wear a special surgical mask, gown

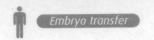

and hat when we got there and that the actual transfer takes place in subdued light in sterile conditions.

In fact, that was mostly old-fashioned horse bollocks.

The magic wand

We arrived at the clinic, went into a room, she lay on a bed and I sat next to her. No funny outfits, no subdued light, and they laughed when I told them about my potential body odours.

It was actually all unnervingly casual.

A kind of serving hatch opened and some teenager in a medical gown handed the specialist what looked like a long plastic stick. Through the hatch we could hear the sound of embryologists having fun. Once again, it felt kind of like being near a sixth-form common room. It wouldn't have surprised me to hear a burst of Judas Priest and get a waft of hash smoke through the hatch.

We were assured that the plastic stick was a catheter with our embryos (we decided to put back two so that there would be slightly more chance of one surviving) on the end. But it really just looked a wand with nothing on the end.

With a certain amount of dexterity, the specialist then poked it up Rosie, suggesting we looked at the screen to see the implantation.

The TV appearance

Expecting to see something rather grand, we stared at a plain black screen of nothing, into which suddenly there appeared a big wand which released a dot.

Just a couple of 'beep' sound effects would have turned the whole thing into a game of Atari Tennis.

Rosie squeezed my hand, partly out of nerves and partly due to the sensitivity of the catheter touching her insides. And that dot on a wand is that. All very brief and hugely underwhelming.

Rosie had also read that clinics invite women to lie still for a while on the bed after the process to encourage the implantation. Also nonsense. This didn't happen in any of our three attempts at IVF.

The photoshoot

Rather bizarrely, the photoshoot seems to be one of the standard parts of the embryo transfer process.

The first time we did IVF we missed out on this at this stage owing to a printer malfunction but the second and third times, just before leaving we were automatically handed a black-and-white Polaroid of our embryonic offspring.

Another great leveller in the creation of a child: the assumption that you would even want a blurred, monochrome photo of a tangled bunch of cells.

Anyway, we were given it. Our child's first portrait. Doesn't it look sweet? Yes. I think it has got my chin.

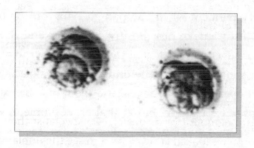

Careless whispers

One other thing.

As warm and happy and positive as you will both try to be going into the clinic after receiving that summoning phone call, this is obviously a very sensitive time emotionally.

You've nearly reached the end of this baby-making journey. You have created an embryo and you are just about to see it placed back into its mum. This means that she will inevitably pick up on the slightest, teensiest bit of negativity from anyone involved that day when you get to the clinic.

Clinics know this, of course they do; they know how tied up IVF is with expectation and anticipation.

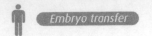

However, they are just human beings doing a job and a fairly scientifically precise job at that.

And maybe the specialist who did the embryo transfer during one of our IVF cycles had had a bad morning, or not enough sleep or had argued with her husband or a colleague or any one of those 283 things that make you a little careless and tetchy at work, but... just as she was handed the plastic wand through the hatch, she commented on Rosie's statistics.

She said something about eggs disintegrating and as she poked the stick up Rosie's front end, she mentioned how maybe there was some other problem that we hadn't encountered that had caused the problem this time, perhaps something like DNA fragmentation in my sperm or something.

Oh no. Oh fuck no.

At the very moment when the patient lying on the bed with her knickers off just wants to hear positive thoughts and good vibes, this woman had inadvertently poked in the poisonous wand of doubt.

She was possibly trying to be helpful, to temper expectations and not give us false hope, to get us to be realistic about our chances and give us other options of exploration, but at that exact moment, when I know what thoughts spun and festered in Rosie's head, I knew that this was *not* helpful.

And I knew what it would mean.

It meant that we would go home after the procedure and at some point during that day Rosie would doubt the survival of the embryos that had been plonked back into her womb. And I knew that if this round of IVF didn't work, it would be my fault.

Yes. It's me.

It was me all along.

And at last we've found out what was wrong. My DNA has fragmented. Of course. That was why it hadn't worked. That is the missing link. My spunk. The woman with the wand said so.

The cost of a careless remark

And thus it came to pass, about six months later, just because of that one comment, I found myself rushing through the rain to a clinic in Harley Street with just minutes to spare, my chest pocket home to yet another tiny plastic pot harbouring several million of my sperm.

Here I was yet again, late and running along a street with a pocketful of wank.

I handed it to a woman at a desk at a cost of several hundred pounds who said it would be sent to a lab in the US, analysed and we would be contacted about the results.

I didn't question how or why it was going across the Atlantic nor quite why I had been given just an hour between wank and delivery when even FedEx will take 24 hours to get it to the States.

But what I did know was that a couple of weeks hence we would get a call or a letter confirming what the law of averages already says: my DNA fragmentation levels were completely normal, we had wasted loads more money and we still didn't know why this IVF thing wasn't working.

You may or may not have a similar situation, but just be prepared.

The people in clinics are just people. They are busy, they have off-days too and the odd, throwaway comment can have costly consequences at this stage.

So begins the wait

Whatever happens, throwaway comments aside, this is a brief, matter-of-fact process.

Almost too matter-of-fact.

She will be up and dressed and going home just 30–45 minutes after she lay down, and every time we did IVF Rosie and I always felt she shouldn't really be standing up so soon in case, at any moment, our embryos might just fall out of her front bottom and splash on to the pavement.

But you've made it to the end. You now have your embryo nestled in her womb, just as it should always have been.

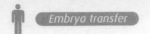

And so begins the two-week wait until she wees on a stick and finds out whether or not you will be parents.

Life's very odd sometimes.

How to survive this stage

* Do whatever you can to keep her upbeat and relaxed. I'm aware that this sentence occurs quite a few times in this book but it can make a huge difference. You know, the power of the mind and all that.

* Remember that you're almost at the end of the whole process. The rest is in the hands of God/the gods/nature*
  (* = delete according to beliefs).

* Be prepared to be underwhelmed. The whole process is brief and pretty routine.

* Also be prepared for the odd thoughtless or impatient member of staff. However hard they may try, they're still human and you're one of probably ten people that day having embryos squirted up them.

* Oh, and be prepared to be confused/underwhelmed by the photos of your embryo. After three attempts we had loads of them and yet somehow they never managed to get its good side.

The consultant says...

The embryo transfer day is, from a doctor's point of view, probably the most critical point of the process to get right. But actually it's the most straightforward part for the patients.

It's vital that the embryos go back in as delicately as possible and in the right place, but for the patient the procedure is no more uncomfortable than a smear test.

Where are you now?

You successfully got through weeks of drugs and egg collection day

*

Your eggs and sperms have mingled

*

You have got some healthy embryos

*

You have been back to the clinic and watched one or two of the embryos being implanted into her womb

*

The medical side of IVF is finally over

*

Now begins the wait to see if it has all worked

*

'Just carry on as normal' is what they will tell you

*

If only it was that simple

10

The two-week wait

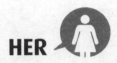

HER

The two-week wait

You've religiously sniffed and injected yourself full of hormones.

You've been scanned, prodded and analysed to within an inch of your life.

You've had a fairly significant operation and got through the ups and downs of fertilisation results.

And you've endured the indignity of a roomful of people peering intensely between your stirruped legs as you've had the most precious thing you've ever created precariously placed back into your womb.

But now you're on your own.

No more doctors or nurses or lab technicians to turn to. No more phone calls or appointments or checks.

It's now just you, your overactive mind and a seemingly endless stretch of time in front of you.

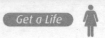

What actually happens

The two-week wait

How long you have to wait depends on when you had your embryo/s put back. Generally, clinics like you to perform a standard urine home pregnancy test (HPT) **at least 14 days** after your egg collection, and often longer. That means…

- If you had embryo transfer on **Day 3** you'll have an **11- to 13-day wait.**
- If you had it on **Day 5** you'll have a **9- to 11-day wait.**

Hence this period is commonly referred to as the two-week wait or the '**2WW**', something you'll see a lot on IVF internet forums.

The drag of time

However long the wait, it feels about ten times longer.

Each day creeps along slowly as you analyse every twinge, cramp and ache that you might (or might not) be feeling. It seems like a peculiar kind of torture that you are helpless to do anything about. All you can do is wait it out, and the idea of test day becomes your sole focus.

However, you are now PUPO, or 'Pregnant Until Proven Otherwise'.

You have every right to presume your treatment has been successful and for me it was a sort of perverse distraction to imagine that I was now pregnant like all my friends, like all those celebrities and women on the train.

I was just like a normal woman at last, about to embark on the most exciting nine months of my life.

I began imagining the little human growing inside me; what would it look like, what would it become, what would it be like to finally be a mother?

Many people would frown at this approach but for me it felt good to fantasise and enjoy the feeling of being (probably/possibly) pregnant at last. At least for these two weeks, anyway.

We IVFers have to take our victories where we can.

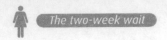

DO NOT TEST EARLY

Of course you will wonder about testing early.

After all, you can sometimes get positive results as early as five or six days after embryo transfer. It may be tempting to take a test, and many do. Often this can be great news if it is positive early, however, if it's negative you run the risk of unnecessarily upsetting yourself as you could still discover that you're actually pregnant a few days later.

So you have to weigh up the possible joy of a positive result with the frustration of a negative result that may not be negative – it just may be too early. If you can bear to wait until it's pretty much definitive, i.e. 14 days since egg collection, then you really should. For your own sanity.

You would not think that was too long to wait, and in terms of the grand scheme of things, of course it isn't. But trust me, it goes tortuously slowly and most people say it is the hardest part of the whole IVF process. I would have to agree.

You'll go particularly mad around Day 5 after transfer (or Day 3 if you've had a five-day transfer), as that's when implantation supposedly could take place.

Some people claim to be able to feel this and some people (though of course not all) have implantation bleeding – a small amount of blood that could just indicate that your clever little embryo/s are bedding in and making themselves comfy in your womb.

Timeline of your embryo

After a Day 3 transfer

1 day post transfer – embryo is growing and developing

2 days post transfer – embryo is now a blastocyst

3 days post transfer – blastocyst hatches out of shell

4 days post transfer – blastocyst attaches to a site on the uterine lining

5 days post transfer – implantation begins as the blastocyst starts to bury itself in the lining

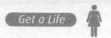
6 days post transfer – implantation process continues and morula buries deeper into the lining

7 days post transfer – morula is completely implanted in the lining and has placenta cells and fetal cells

8 days post transfer – placenta cells begin to secrete HCG in the blood

9 days post transfer – more HCG is produced as fetus develops

10 days post transfer – more HCG is produced as fetus develops

11 days post transfer – HCG levels are now high enough to be immediately detected on HPT

After a Day 5 transfer

1 day post transfer – blastocyst hatches out of shell

2 days post transfer – blastocyst attaches to a site on the uterine lining

3 days post transfer – implantation begins, as the blastocyst begins to bury into the lining

4 days post transfer – implantation process continues and morula buries deeper into the lining

5 days post transfer – morula is completely implanted in the lining and has placenta cells and fetal cells

6 days post transfer – placenta cells begin to secrete HCG in the blood

7 days post transfer – more HCG is produced as fetus develops

8 days post transfer – more HCG is produced as fetus develops

9 days post transfer – HCG levels are now high enough to be immediately detected on HPT

Misleading signs

As time goes on you'll be looking out for pregnancy signs and again over-analysing all of them. Are my boobs sore? Do I feel a bit sick? Did I just feel a twinge down there?

The truth is, of course, that you probably won't feel much at all at this very early stage of pregnancy, but that won't stop your imagination running wild. Just try to remember that your mind is a very powerful tool and can invent all sorts of physical symptoms that don't really exist.

Rather helpfully, progesterone can mimic both PMT and pregnancy symptoms: sore boobs, the need to urinate more frequently and of course mood swings. Oh, and constipation is one of the most common side effects too.

This means that you feel you are either very pregnant or about to have the worst period of your life. As I mentioned before, progesterone is a cruel, cruel drug.

More about it below.

Don't be over-cautious

You'll also probably find yourself taking all sorts of unnecessary precautions.

I was terrified of baths and hot-water bottles in case I scrambled the embryos. You probably won't want to do any heavy lifting, drink alcohol, have sex or eat soft cheese, just in case.

The clinics generally advise you to get on with life as normal but to limit certain activities (like swimming, marathon running and skydiving) but it depends how cautious you are as to what you want to do.

Some people will advise 48-hour bed rest after your embryo transfer while others suggest going back to work and getting on with life as normal. I did something between the two and took a couple of days off to watch films and chill out before going back to work, which at least made the days go quicker.

It really is a very testing time and you will find it really hard to concentrate on anything else.

After all you've been though with the IVF procedure the thought of a negative result looms like a black cloud creeping in over the distant horizon.

Try not to let it in, just yet.

How you will feel physically

Meanwhile, you are still dealing with the physical recovery from the IVF procedures.

Your ovaries may still feel a bit swollen from egg collection and if you're unlucky you may have a touch of OHSS where you're very bloated and uncomfortable.

OHSS is when your empty follicles start filling up with fluid, which can lead to swelling, pain, shortness of breath and, in extreme cases, needs hospitalisation.

Having said this, OHSS can get worse with pregnancy so if you do start to feel ill with it then there is an upside, as it could mean you are actually pregnant. At the first sign of symptoms you should see your doctor and do an early pregnancy test to get confirmation.

More on progesterone

You thought you'd finished with all the drugs but actually now you are taking some of the most horrible ones of all – progesterone. Usually this is supplied in pessary form for you to administer yourself either up the vagina or up the bum. Delightful.

Progesterone is needed to keep the womb lining thick and healthy to support a pregnancy and if you're pregnant you'll take it for a short time beyond your positive result, sometimes up to the crucial 12-week mark.

Non-IVF conceptions produce this hormone naturally, but after the drugs of IVF have mucked up your system you need the help of artificial progesterone to make sure you have enough of the hormone in your system.

So it's a very important drug to take, but it's horrible. Not only is it a messy pessary (panty liners are compulsory unless you want to ruin all your nicest knickers), but it also seems to mimic the PMT symptoms you would feel in a normal cycle.

It does for me anyway. It makes me feel moody, depressed and anxious. A really great combination when you already have good reason to be going fairly mad.

However, there's not much you can do about all this. You've got to

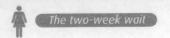

keep taking it so you just need to accept that it will mess with your hormones a bit and try to find other ways to get happy.

What happened to us

How I got through the two-week wait

I turned to a number of different coping techniques to get me though the two-week wait.

Obviously different things work for different people but for me it was vital to get some emotional support.

Things I did:

- I saw an acupuncturist to help with blood flow and supposedly encourage implantation.

- I had some reflexology sessions as a relaxing treat for me (I am a firm believer in pampering myself in times of stress).

- Probably the greatest help during this time was having some phone sessions with a hypnotherapist. I needed to think positively and start 'connecting' with my embryos. Even if I was heading for a negative result, there was no harm in thinking positively about them for the short time they were on board. That's the thing about IVF, you just have to have hope, no matter how much the odds are stacked against you.

- Of course, it was also good to schedule in some nice outings and visits with family and friends. However, only see people you really love being with. You will feel very vulnerable at this stage and there's no point wasting your time with anyone who isn't sympathetic and positive (this is generally a good rule in life anyway). It's also good if you can see people you can talk to about IVF as that is all that will be on your mind anyway.

However you approach it and however long and tedious it seems, the two-week wait WILL eventually pass and you will reach the end of this tortuous period.

By the time you've got to the eve of test day, you'll be wishing you could stay in your blissful ignorance forever – at least that way there's still a possibility of being pregnant.

But test you must, as you approach the last hurdle of the IVF assault course.

How to survive this stage

* Remember, there's nothing you can actually do now to influence the outcome. You can't take control of this situation, you just need to let go and let your body do its work.

* Take some time to chill out at home if you can – at least for the first couple of days. Watch bad films and enjoy a good laugh or even a little weep – it's good to let out all those conflicting emotions.

* Remember that when you are weeping uncontrollably or shouting angrily at your partner, or even feeling sore boobs and nausea, it's probably due to the progesterone rather than PMT or pregnancy. Progesterone has a lot to answer for.

* Schedule in nice things to do and sympathetic people to see. Book a facial or a haircut, or a cinema evening with your friends. Pamper yourself; you've been through a lot.

* Limit who you tell. All you need right now is endless texts and calls from people who are anxious to know the outcome. Tell people who know you've been through a cycle that you will call them when you have news and they're not to ask in the meantime.

* Schedule in time to 'obsess' about your symptoms. You'll want to be on the internet and comparing notes with others all day long but try

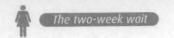

to limit the time you do this. Set aside just 20 minutes a day to look up or think about whatever it is that is bothering you. Then when things pop up you can remind yourself to check them out later rather than immediately going straight to Dr Google.

* Make a date with your partner for the night of your pregnancy test. If it is positive, you can celebrate together. If it is negative, you can have a good cry and start talking about what to do next.

* Have an idea of how you're going to cope if it is a negative result. Will you plan another cycle soon, do some more tests or give yourself a break? It's good to have a plan B up your sleeve if the worst happens on test day.

* If you feel anxious or unsupported, or if just have questions, call your clinic. You've invested a lot of time and perhaps money in these people and you are still under their care. They'll want to know if you have any concerns and they should give you support when you phone in your test results.

* Don't test early. Don't test early. DON'T TEST EARLY. It's simply not worth it. Be patient and you'll at least have a definitive answer.

HIM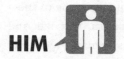

The two-week wait

You've made it.

It seems like ages ago that you first both talked about doing IVF but now you've finally done it.

All that waiting and testing and wanking and probing and stress and fear and blame and drugs and pain is finally over.

All you need to do now is just carry on as you were and wait for her to do a pregnancy test in about a fortnight. Piece of piss.

Er, no.

What actually happens

Women v Men

Imagine that, for about the last 20 years of your life, you'd really wanted something.

You'd wanted it quite a lot initially but with each passing year you'd wanted it more and more.

In recent years you could barely control how much you wanted this thing. You couldn't describe what it meant to you, you just knew you were incomplete without this thing.

Even worse, you are surrounded by TV and magazines and newspapers telling you that time is running out for you and you'd better have this thing soon or it will be too late. And if you don't have one you will be a shadow of the person you are now, a lonely failure.

Your body is telling you the same thing, too.

It's releasing hormones into your brain telling you YOU MUST HAVE THIS THING as that is what you are here to do.

And suddenly everywhere you look other people have one of these things and you still don't. In fact, they often have more than one. And your friends have got them too. And some of them didn't even really want one but they've got one anyway. And you STILL don't.

But then you find out that there is a medical procedure you can have that might – just might – make it possible for you to have one of these things.

You know the odds are stacked against you and you know that you might have to pay an enormous amount of money to have the procedure, even with the probability that it won't work. You know that none of this makes any sense to anyone but you, but you decide to do it anyway.

And then, several months and a lot of unpleasant physical investigation and drugs later, you have completed the procedure and you have seen on a TV screen a doctor plant the seed of the thing you've wanted so much all this time inside you.

You are then told to go home and just hope that it stays there and grows and you'll know in about two weeks whether it has worked and whether you will finally have the thing you've wanted for as long as you can remember.

Well that, that is what the two-week wait is like for a woman.

In fact, it's probably like that multiplied by a factor of 762.

Probably.

I don't know.

And neither do you.

Because we're not built like that.

But I do know that *you* can just go home and carry on as normal but inside *her* is a feeling like no other.

What she will be like

She will be tired and a little fragile after all the events and procedures of the last five weeks, that's pretty obvious.

Lots of rest and warm baths and nice meals and good films can help with that, but the greatest battle – as it is with all of IVF – is with the mind.

Her mind will not switch off and will feed her unhelpful messages.

She knows she has to think of something else and there's nothing more she can do but her mind will be telling her that the IVF has worked.

Or it hasn't.

Every single twinge and ache and pain and specks of blood in her pants and soreness in her boobs will be telling her the same thing.

She will also be taking a drug (I promise it's the last one) to help thicken her womb lining and make it all nice and warm and snug for any visiting embryos.

The drug is progesterone. It's produced naturally in non-IVF conception but because all those IVF powders and sniffing drugs have mucked with her system she has to take it now.

Rather delightfully, it's a pessary which is taken up her bum or vagina and, rather helpfully, it mimics the symptoms of both pregnancy *and* PMT. That means she might actually genuinely feel physically pregnant when she's not and she'll be as moody as a witch.

Chuck that into the whirlwind of psychology that's going on anyway and you'll understand why many women (including Rosie) find this stage of IVF the hardest bit. Without the right approach this fortnight could unleash a volcano of boiling shit on a previously happy relationship.

What progesterone actually does
... just in case you want to know

- During the menstrual cycle, when an egg is released from the ovary at ovulation (about Day 14), the remnants of the ovarian follicle release progesterone.

- Progesterone prepares the body for pregnancy just in case the egg is fertilised.

- If it is fertilised, progesterone stimulates the growth of blood vessels supplying the womb.

- It prepares the tissue lining of the uterus to allow the fertilised egg to implant.

- In the early stages of pregnancy, progesterone is essential for supporting the embryo and establishing the placenta.

- Once the placenta is established it then takes over progesterone production.

- The level of progesterone steadily rises throughout pregnancy.

Source: yourhormones.info

What happened to us

The first time

The first time we did IVF Rosie knew what she should be doing but just couldn't actually do it.

She knew the best thing to do was to keep busy and take her mind off the whole thing as best she could.

She did acupuncture and hypnotherapy and knew she should be going for massages and seeing friends but nothing could take her mind off it.

For several days after embryo transfer she just lay around the house under a blanket, either sleeping or watching telly. She was knackered, of course, but also deep down she assumed she should barely exert herself for fear of jogging the embryos out of place.

As I explained earlier, owing to my debacle in the wank booth, the embryos had a hugely reduced chance of survival anyway, but Rosie had wanted to just be and feel pregnant for so long she cocooned herself in psychological bubble wrap, did nothing whatsoever that might jeopardise their safety and urged the 14 days to go quicker.

The second and third times

The second and third times we did IVF Rosie was a little wiser and tried to carry on more normally, but the mind is a delicate little sponge at times.

Again, she knew she should see friends but she couldn't bear the questioning and the faux sympathy. Friends – even actual nice ones – want to be nice and sympathise but really unless you've been through IVF you have no idea what the frigging hell it is like.

She also learnt after the failed first time to limit the number of people she told that she was doing IVF. This is rather easier said than done – particularly if the IVF drugs do have side effects and she's going to work feeling like a mad old shitbag.

The early test

The other problem is that even though the clinic will (rightly) tell her not to do a pregnancy test until at least 14 days after egg collection day, it is, again, so much easier said than done. Not least because even at 11 days it might show up positive.

But I promise you, you must try to stop her doing it.

That obviously doesn't mean trying to stop her weeing completely at around the 11-day mark, as that can just result in her bladder exploding and is probably against the law. Just try to stop her weeing on those little sticks.

It is incredibly hard.

Each of these 14 days seems interminable. The whole thing is a shitty mess of anticipation and rough timing. But patience is key.

Even though we're a pack of drunk, lazy, lecherous morons these two weeks will make you realise how lucky you are to be a man.

I thanked God each day for my testicles, as unsightly and ludicrous as they quite clearly are.

How to survive this stage

* Try to empathise with what she's going through. It's impossible, really, but try.

* Do anything you can to try to take her mind off the whole thing. That's impossible too but even momentarily or a few hours can make a difference.

* Limit who you tell about IVF at this stage. It saves a whole heap of crappy faux sentimentality if the process doesn't work.

* Definitely make sure she doesn't just lie around under a blanket. Rosie realised this the second time. There's a great rule of nature that if the embryos are healthy and meant to turn into babies they will. Usual activity such as walking, etc., will have no effect. Only activities such as bungee-jumping, kick-boxing or armed combat should probably be ruled out. Or at least postponed.

* Prohibit her (yes, I know, as if she'll pay a blind bit of notice to anything you say) or at least try to stop her from doing an early pregnancy test. Remind her you are 50 per cent of this baby-making process. That line goes down *really* well at this stage...

The consultant says...

My main advice is to do as little or as much as you need to so you can stay as stress-free as you can.

Try to live life as normally as you can.

Work, exercise, sex, lifting, etc., is not going to change the genetics of the embryo so just try to do whatever you need to ensure that you don't end up spending 24 hours a day thinking about it.

Where are you now?

You have been back to the clinic and seen your embryo/s being
implanted into the womb

*

The doctors at the clinic have finished their bit

*

You have managed to get through a truly testing couple of
weeks hoping that the whole procedure has worked

*

Now comes the actual testing time

11

Test day

HER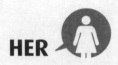

Test day

So this is it, the moment you've all been waiting for.

The moment of truth.

D-Day.

Or, rather, T-Day.

Call it what you will, it is as scary as your A-level exam results day and as important as your wedding day.

What actually happens

I always thought it odd that you were left to perform such an important test on your own.

Generally in the UK you are just given a bog-standard HPT (home pregnancy test) and are expected to do the standard urine test like every other potential pregnant woman out there. No special treatment, no clinician checking your results. This always felt a bit of an anticlimax to me.

In the United States you go into the clinic for a blood test to measure

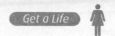

the levels of the pregnancy hormone HCG in the blood, which is thought to be more accurate than the levels in urine. That always felt like it would be a more satisfactory option – at least you're in a clinic with medical support around you and not just at home perched unceremoniously over a toilet.

A bit about HCG (human chorionic gonadotropin)

HCG is the pregnancy hormone which becomes present in your urine and in your blood as soon as you become pregnant.

- A pregnancy that is developing in the womb normally will result in the levels of HCG hormone in the blood approximately doubling every 48 hours.

- A level that is continually decreasing by approximately 50% generally indicates that a pregnancy is miscarrying or failing to develop.

- Levels that remain 'static' can indicate an ectopic pregnancy or an early pregnancy in the womb that is no longer developing normally.

Source: www.hampshirehospitals.nhs.uk/media/16264/hcg_info_leaflet_march2010.pdf

---

Before the test

When to do it

You will probably not have slept much the night before and there lies the first of your many dilemmas.

If you are up worrying and need a wee you have to weigh up whether to wee and hopefully go back to sleep or lie there holding on to your wee so you can test with 'first morning urine' which will be the most undiluted and therefore give you the most accurate result. 'FMU' is ideally what you want to test with.

Or, of course, you can get up and wee AND test in the middle of the night but then you need to decide how you're going to cope with the result at three o'clock in the morning.

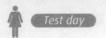

You are not going to go back to sleep afterwards whatever it is and your partner may not be so happy to stay up and celebrate/commiserate with you at that time of the morning.

So, the first decision you need to make is when you are going to test and then stick by it. I always held out until about 7 a.m., when I could stand it no more.

Which test are you going to use?

The second decision is what test/tests are you going to use?

You may get given a pregnancy test by your clinic or just told to buy one from the chemist.

Although they are testing the same thing – the level of HCG, the pregnancy hormone, in the urine – all tests are not the same.

Some will offer you the 'smiley face' pregnant or not pregnant icon whereas others give you a line or a cross to denote a positive result. If you've been trying for some time you proabably will have invested in some 'internet cheapies' – those thin strips that are pretty basic.

Bear in mind that you'll probably want to do a couple of tests as it will be hard to rely on any one result, so it's good to have some backup tests up your sleeve so you can double check (although try not to do more than three otherwise you really are wasting your time and money).

Also, I recommend taking a sample of urine in a small pot so you can do a few tests on the same bit of 'first morning urine' rather than see it get flushed down the toilet.

Some pregnancy tests just say to wee on to the absorbent stick bit but once that wee has gone, it's gone, and your next wee may not be so potent and you're going to want to do some more tests with the good wee so make sure you harvest it. I know this all sounds mental, but trust me.

Plan the rest of the day

The third decision to make is what you are going to do that day.

Are you going to go to work? Is that really sensible if you get a negative result? Can you switch off your emotions that easily and get on with your

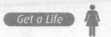
job or are you going to need some time to process the result, whatever it is?

I always booked a day off work during all three cycles as I wanted to avoid having a crying fit in the work toilets at all costs.

The key moment

So, you're there, pregnancy test in hand, urine sample at the ready and you now have to take the plunge and put the two together.

I have always been near hysterical at this point. Shaking and sweating like I'm about to be sentenced to life imprisonment.

Let's face it, your bathroom toilet is not usually a place for high drama but in this instance it really is a life-changing moment and you have so many of your life's hopes and dreams riding on it, so it's not that surprising you're going to freak out a little. Just try not to drop the wee or the test down the toilet.

Of course, once you've dipped that stick into the wee you've then got to wait for a good five minutes for it to 'season'. As if you haven't waited enough.

That's what infertility is all about: waiting.

By now, though, you will have become a master of patience and you must muster all your coping techniques to just get through this last push before you finally find out if this whole thing has been worth it or not.

Yes, it all comes down to that moment in the bathroom.

Is that a line?

You look at the test stick and with all your might you will there to be a little pink line.

Is that a line? Or is that a shadow? It's nowhere near as dark as the test line but could it actually be the faint beginnings of a positive result?

You will end up peering at the stick, holding it up to the light, taking it to a window, looking at it from all different angles and wondering if your eyes are about to pop out of your head and your heart out of your mouth.

Of course, you may now want to do another of your pregnancy tests, using a different brand to compare and contrast.

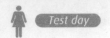

Whatever you see you will probably end up doubting it. It's now time to wake up your partner and get them involved in the whole farcical situation. Hopefully a voice of rationality will be able to determine the truth of the situation and finally confirm what you already in your heart of hearts know, whether that be positive or negative.

Home pregnancy tests: dos and don'ts

DO

- Test with FMU – first morning urine

- Check the expiry date (on the inner wrapping of the test and not just the box). Yes, they do go off

- Buy pregnancy tests online and in bulk – much cheaper than the ones in shops

- Collect your urine in a little pot (ramekins are perfect) so that you can retest using the same FMU

DON'T

- Re-use tests. Once wee-ed on they become invalid.

- Just rely on one brand of test on test day. Have a couple of different ones to double-check your result.

- Keep re-checking the tests. Most manufacturers say to discard it after ten minutes as after that odd shadows and lines can appear that will give misleading results.

- Test early, especially as your trigger drug contains HCG – the same hormone used to detect pregnancy on home pregnancy tests so you may get a false positive

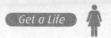

What happened to us

I've had both outcomes.

The first time was resoundingly negative and the immense sinking feeling when it became clear that the stick was going to stay spitefully blank was intense.

I had to just crawl back into bed, tell Richard and try to sleep off the disappointment before I faced the world and started spreading the news and trying to deal with the outcome.

More on that in the next chapter.

But I've also had the joy of seeing a positive line. Twice.

The first time, despite doubting it for a very long time, I finally believed in the little pink shadow and felt confident enough to wake Richard up by shouting 'I'M PREGNANT' in a manner wholly inappropriate for 7 a.m.

Of course, that pregnancy was not to be (see my miscarriage diary in Chapter 14), so the second time I saw a positive test (during our third IVF attempt) I reacted in a far more measured way.

I was still delighted, of course, but probably more relieved than anything.

The thought of our third cycle failing would have been a little too much to bear, so to see a positive was truly amazing, although not worthy of the ecstasy I'd felt before.

At least that meant it wasn't the end of the road just yet and we still had some of that most important of IVF emotions: hope.

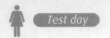

How to survive this stage

* Prepare. Buy your tests. Cheap ones or expensive ones with the smiley face – at least someone gets to be happy.

* Plan your wees. Decide when you're going to test in the morning and work backwards. You'll need a nice stock of urine so make sure you leave it a good six or seven hours before THE wee.

* Discuss with your partner whether they will do the test with you, look at the result for you or leave you to it.

* Book the day off work and clear your diary for a few days – be realistic about how a negative test might affect you.

* Wee in a pot so you can retest and don't have to wait until you need to wee again.

* Get your clinic details ready to phone in with the result.

* Take a deep breath before you dip that stick. Yes, your hand is shaking, yes, it feels like your head is about to burst but really, get a grip, woman. And preferably a firm one.

* Once wee has met stick, leave it (carefully) on the side and walk away for five minutes. Don't torture yourself waiting for the lines to appear, check it when it's actually done.

* Have your mum/sister/a good friend ready on the other end of the phone to celebrate/commiserate with. It will be early so you'll need to pick someone who isn't rushing off to work.

HIM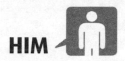

Test day

Oh, come on.

Surely the simple act of a woman weeing on a little plastic stick really doesn't warrant its own chapter, does it?

Yes, it really does.

This isn't just a wee. It's the wee of wees. The most important wee she might ever do. A wee that signifies victory or defeat.

What actually happens

Now, I know you won't pay much attention to any of this.

I know this because Rosie explained it to me during our first attempt at IVF and I didn't pay attention.

But I assure you, it's worth knowing even though it really is utterly ridiculous.

You see, it's all about the timing of her wee and the type of testing kit, apparently.

All testing kits are testing for the same thing, the level of a hormone called HCG. No, I don't know what it stands for either and by this stage I was pretty cocking sick of acronyms. But they announce the result in different ways, depending on how expensive they are.

A plastic stick to wee on

By now you probably know what a pregnancy testing kit looks like (our bathroom cupboards were full of them) but in case you don't (and I really didn't until we started this whole baby-making business) they generally look like this:

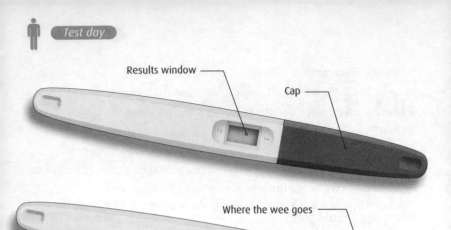

Results window

Cap

Where the wee goes

There are fancier versions available but essentially it is just a little plastic stick that she pisses on and it shows up a little line if it's positive.

Generally they all do the same thing – the cheap, thin testing sticks or the chunky plastic ones from what I learnt after three attempts. She will know this, of course, and you might do too, depending on how much money she's spent and how much urinating on little sticks she's done in the last few years.

How they show if she's pregnant

They indicate pregnancy in different ways.

- A **pinky red line** will appear in the little indicator box.

- A **cross** will denote a positive response.

- A **smiley face** icon appears.

Yes. Honestly.

For the amount of money they cost and for what they are being used to indicate I think I would want a bit more than that. Perhaps a little trumpet fanfare, or a car alarm, or the *Family Fortunes* 'ee-aww' noise. Or, to diffuse a bit of the tension from the occasion, maybe a Vic 'n' Bob *Shooting Stars*-style 'Oovavoo'.

A smiley face just smacks of a text from a teenager. This is the creation of human life we're talking about, you tacky fuckers.

When she should wee

The timing of the wee is also key. (An unintentional rhyme.) It needs to be the big, early morning wee of that fourteenth day.

Trouble is, she will be a tad nervous and probably won't sleep the night before. She may want to wee in the middle of the night, not unusually, and then she's in the middle of a urinal gamble.

She knows the wee for the test needs to be the most undiluted, so does she wee in the middle of the night and hope there's enough for the morning? Or hold it in until about 7 a.m. Yes. This is what your love life has now become. Quite literally a load of piss.

What happened to us

The first time we did IVF, Rosie didn't sleep at all the night before the test.

Despite my best empathising (which, even by the International Empathy Scale was scoring much higher than usual), I couldn't possibly comprehend what she was going through and I woke up when she went to the bathroom. She seemed to be in there ages and it was only ages later that I realised why.

She'd been advised to take a sample of urine in a small pot so she could do a few tests on the same load of early morning wee. So to do that, well, you can probably imagine the logistics.

Unfortunately, by this stage Rosie was almost unable to control her hands or arms. Unparalleled quantities of apprehension and hysteria had resulted in paroxysms of fear.

Because this was the moment.

The moment. The yes or no.

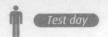

She'd seen them put an embryo back and this was the moment when she would find out whether or not she was pregnant for the first time in her life.

And there was the wait.

Of course there was the wait.

You'd expect nothing else by this stage. It's what IVF is good at – apart from lots of acronyms – waiting.

The little plastic stick wasn't immediate in its response. It took a few minutes to absorb its discharge and make up its mind. So she didn't know if she hadn't left it long enough or whether it just hadn't worked.

What happens when it's negative

Then there's the issue of that little plastic stick remaining stubbornly blank. Perhaps she hadn't done it properly. Perhaps it was a dud. So she did a few to double and triple and quadruple check. And still no line.

That first time I knew the result before she told me, simply by the way the bathroom light was turned off and the way she got into bed. She was shaking and crying and quietly managed to squeeze out the words 'I'm not pregnant'.

There is then the issue of what happens to the rest of the day/week.

Rosie was pretty savvy on each of our three attempts and always took the day off work on test day. Even on the second and third times when she had a positive result. It just saves a day of intrusion and distraction.

I'm sure your partner will do the same. It's a very good idea. I'm not sure how Rosie would have coped that first time.

Anyway, there's more about all this in Chapter 12.

What happens when it's positive

Of course, the second time we did IVF, Rosie also double- and triple- and quadruple-checked her piss-sticks.

This time it was because she couldn't quite comprehend that there did actually appear to be a line/smiley face/trumpet fanfare.

The second time we did IVF I knew the result before she told me by the sound of the woman who married me screaming with uncontrollable, maniacal joy.

My expertise in all matters urinal was naturally called in to check the situation and there on the plastic wee stick, the stick that had been resolutely blank and unlined for years, was indeed the faintest of pink lines. Barely visible, but there.

It became slightly more prominent, redder, a few hours later and was then unmistakeable.

For the first time in more than a third of a century on the planet, Rosie was pregnant.

Eight weeks later we would realise the jubilation was premature when an ultrasound scan revealed Rosie had had a miscarriage (more on what that is actually like in Chapter 14).

Learning from mistakes

So on the third time we did IVF and the wee stick showed the faint red line, Rosie's joy was more tempered. Make no mistake, she was triumphant, but it was measured. Good old life and its clever way of making you learn from previous behaviour.

And on this third time there was the usual sleepless night for Rosie, the grand deliberation over when to wee and the hand spasms as she tested in the bathroom.

BUT this time there was not the leap on the bed.

Just relief.

Relief that the second time hadn't been a freak result. And relief that this wasn't the end of her dream and she'd been given another chance.

As we'd learnt that second time, there is more waiting until you go for a 'viability' scan to check that the test stick hasn't lied, but for now this little pink line is the greatest hurdle and the odds in the casino of life are back in your favour.

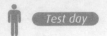

How to survive this stage

* It will be impossible, you know that, but just try the best you can to empathise with what she's going through. The whole process is absurd, crude and unfair.

* Do what you can to make sure she doesn't wee on her stick before the 14-day mark. (What an odd sentence that is...)

* If she does test early and gets a negative result, try to keep her hopes up. A negative can still be a positive a couple of days later.

* Make sure she doesn't go to work on this day, whatever the result.

* The second time we did IVF I remember hearing Rosie upstairs for a couple of hours phoning ALL her friends and family, deliriously shouting 'IT'S WORKED!!! I'M PREGNANT' and regretting it a few weeks later when the scan proved otherwise. Again, be careful who you tell and who she tells at this early stage.

* Both negative and positive results are hard in different ways, so there's more on how to survive each of them in the next two chapters.

The consultant says...

If you are testing at home make sure you test with the 'first catch' urine of the morning because it's going to be the most concentrated.

Try not to test too early because you might get unnecessarily disappointed.

As for pregnancy testing kits, the cheap ones are fine – they are all so accurate, don't stress about which one you buy.

Where are you now?

You have managed to get through the
gruelling two-week wait

*

You have also finally done a pregnancy test
If it was negative, do not despair

*

Hopefully the next chapter will have some words of help

*

If it was positive, feel free to skip to Chapter 13
for some advice on what to do now

12

How to cope with a negative result

HER

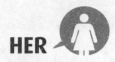

How to cope with a negative result

Seeing the stubbornly stark white test stick is probably nothing new for you, I had seen that many, many times before on my natural cycles, but this one really kicks hard to the stomach.

This one isn't just something to bin, process and move on from quickly into the next cycle. This one feels like a real statement.

It says 'even when you turn to the experts and even when you have the sperm and the egg turn into an actual living embryo, you still can't manage it'.

It will leave you panicking and thinking, 'what now?'

There are some tips at the end of this chapter on how to cope and hopefully they will relieve some of the panic.

What happened to us

After getting a negative result this was my first thought:

If IVF fails, what do I do next?

I had always thought of IVF as the last resort but now I needed a new last resort and I didn't know what it might be. Donor eggs? Donor sperm? Adoption? Childlessness?

All those thoughts rushed through my head in the ten seconds it took me to walk upstairs with my negative pregnancy test in hand to show Richard.

I remember crawling back into bed (I think it was still pretty early) and wanting to stay there forever.

Spreading the bad news

I didn't sleep, of course.

I knew I had to get up and tell all the people I had foolishly told I was testing that day.

Calling my parents was hard. They were as upset as me but tried to be upbeat for my sake.

Friends were, of course, hugely supportive, but ultimately they were not able to have an in-depth conversation about infertility on their way to work. So Richard and I trundled through the day, feeling upset and not really sure what to do about it.

Another attempt?

My default position was to get on the internet and start looking up what to do next.

I devoured the forums and started investigating new clinics we could try. We had been lucky to get that first round on the NHS but now, if we were to try again, we'd be looking at paying for a private clinic. It meant a massive bill but at least we had a lot of choice.

The average cost of a basic no-frills IVF cycle where we live is around £5–7K. Could we even afford that?

We could go with somewhere local or one of the top London clinics or even look at going abroad and making a strange sort of fertility holiday of it – like a spa break but with less massage and hot towels and more needles and anaesthesia.

Richard wasn't quite as ready to jump ahead to the next step as I was and I think that's fairly normal.

Men process things in different ways and he probably wanted to let the dust settle before manically planning our next move. But for me that was the only way I could cope.

I needed a new plan of action, then at least I could regain a little bit of hope. Aahhh, hope.

Maybe this round failed because of the delayed fertilisation, or maybe the consultants or the lab weren't the best but if we were paying to go one of the top clinics then surely things would work next time? Surely?

So for me, planning the next cycle was a good coping technique.

That can be a slippery slope, though. As you probably know, IVF can be really addictive and when you hear about couples who've done it seven, eight or nine times you can see how easily that could happen.

The emotional impact

As the days went on I gradually got back to normal but I still had some embarrassing moments. Like when I would be walking around a car park on the phone to my mum saying how I was feeling fine and then would hang up and start crying. Crying in car parks is never a good thing, is it?

I just felt sad, really. Really, really sad.

It was stupid to have expected IVF to work first time and I knew I shouldn't have placed all my hopes and expectations on it, but I did and just felt so let down that it had failed and that I was still 'infertile', still not pregnant and still no further forward.

The impact on our relationship

I'd tried the supposedly failsafe, expensive, invasive, scientific technique and still no joy. How long was this going to go on? How long could I go on doing it and how long would Richard?

That was another problem – I'm a determined (aka stubborn) old sod and I had in the back of my mind that I would keep trying and doing IVF for as long as it took to achieve my goal, but I knew Richard didn't share that plan.

He had found this first cycle and the 'incident in the booth' so traumatic that I knew he wouldn't want to keep going forever.

Plus there was the cost and hassle of it all and having our lives on hold in the meantime.

Injecting drugs and sniffing hormones is not conducive to a happy, normal, carefree life. We did talk about it and I knew that he didn't want to turn into one of those couples who did IVF ten times, wasting years of their lives and tens of thousands of pounds on it (which we definitely did not have), but I couldn't bring myself to put a time limit on it – that just made me panic more.

So we sort of left that disharmony floating in the air a bit and hoped that we wouldn't have to ever make those decisions about when to stop. The thought of stopping, without having a baby, was just too much to bear.

The physical impact

Of course, that's all just the emotional stuff – there was also the recovery from the physical trial my body had been through.

After all, it had been messed with for weeks, being pumped full of strange hormones and then given a potential human being to play with.

As soon as you phone in to your clinic with a negative result they tell you to stop taking progesterone as your body no longer needs to support a potential pregnancy. So begins your hormonal system's arduous task of getting back into balance.

It can take weeks for your cycle to get back to normal following an IVF cycle, which can be very depressing, especially if you want to get back in the saddle (so to speak) pretty quickly.

Clinics generally like you to have one whole natural cycle after a failed cycle before going again, so you have to wait for your period to start. And because of all the drugs this can sometimes be a long wait.

I was fairly lucky and my cycle returned relatively quickly but some people wait months.

I think a course of acupuncture can really help to regulate things and get your cycle back to normal. That first period, when it comes, is bittersweet. At least it means you are back to normal and can start to try again – either with IVF or naturally – but of course it is also the definitive sign that you're definitely not pregnant, there's been no miraculous mistake, no hidden baby growing secretly and undetected. And yes, even though it's madness you will have been thinking that there is.

The horrible truth is that you have to face the fact that this IVF cycle just hasn't worked.

As much as it might feel like it at the time, it isn't the end of the world and below are a few tips on how to get through it.

What went wrong?

There is usually no obvious explanation as to why embryos fail to develop in the womb but one of the following may be relevant:

- **Embryos have a reduced chance of implanting** – the egg may not have matured properly, or may not have divided as it should after fertilisation.

- **Chromosome problems** – many embryos that look healthy have faulty chromosomes – the structures inside cells that contain genes and control how the cell works and what it does.

- **Poor blood flow to the uterus** – even if there is nothing wrong with the quality of the embryos, If circulation to the urerus is poor you have less chance of getting pregnant and a greater chance of miscarriage if you do conceive.

Source: www.hfea.gov.uk/78.html

How to survive this stage

* Remember, you did nothing wrong. After embryo transfer, there is really nothing you can do to influence the embryo implanting successfully.

* Remind yourself that this is nature doing its job – the embryo didn't survive for a reason.

* Take time to grieve – schedule in a dressing-gown day (or two).

* Don't tell everyone when you are testing, be vague or you will get loads of concerned texts that might tip you over the edge.

* Don't feel you have to tell the people who do know straight away – they will understand that you will let them know when you're ready.

* Make a plan of what to do next, research your options.

* Have a conversation beforehand with your partner about how far you are going to go in your quest to have a child so there are no surprises when you are in slight hysterical panic mode.

* Do some nice things you couldn't do if you were pregnant – get drunk, eat your bodyweight in soft cheese.

* Don't hate your body for being crap. Nurture and heal your body for what it's been through. Book a massage or facial, go on holiday. Just pamper yourself.

* Only see the people who cheer you up and don't waste time on others, though be aware that some people just don't know what to say, so they say nothing. It's not very helpful, but don't take offence.

HIM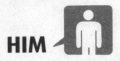

How to cope with a negative result

I'm putting this bit in purely as a coping mechanism as this stage can be really hard on a relationship.

So many of our feelings about IVF are along the lines of 'if we knew then what we know now' and this stage is particularly true.

You've seen them put an embryo into her womb.

You've watched it on a TV screen.

You've even got a photo of it.

Not unreasonably, therefore, you expect it has worked.

But when that pregnancy stick refuses to show a line or a smiley face, her world, and therefore yours, slightly collapses underneath you.

What happened to us

Even though we knew that our first attempt at IVF was pretty doomed by my seedless shenanigans in the Wank Booth, incredibly, by test day, we still believed that it might have worked.

Mostly because Rosie so wanted it to work and probably because we didn't know any better.

And all that despite the chances we were given at the outset.

We'd seen the embryos being embedded in Rosie's womb, she had felt twinges and swollen knockers. She had felt a bit sick and she'd told friends of hers who had babies about all this and they told her what a good sign all that was and that she really was almost certainly pregnant.

But that morning when she crawled back into bed, shaking and in tears, just able to say the words 'I'm not pregnant... it hasn't worked', I wasn't aware how bad the next few weeks and months would be and really what 'it hasn't worked' meant this time.

How she feels (probably)

By the time you do IVF your partner will have wee-ed on lots of plastic sticks. Not hundreds but very possibly dozens.

Each month it may have been disheartening and slightly soul-destroying but that was nothing compared to this blank stick.

To her, this one said that even after all those tests and drugs and embryologists and specialists and all that medical advancement, even with people actually ENGINEERING your eggs and sperms to make embryos and even after you actually saw them put an embryo into your womb, even then you still can't get pregnant.

It really exposes the stark reality of childlessness for the first time.

The unspoken possibility

What's particularly stupid is that after the embryos were plonked into Rosie's womb we never discussed the – very real – possibility that it hadn't worked.

Neither of us dared to raise it. Not at all.

The whole awful two-week wait was so artificially imbued with positive thoughts that the possibility of failure was sealed in a lead-lined container and buried.

We knew before even starting IVF that we only had a 30 per cent chance of 'live birth' (that lovely phrase). That meant there was a 70 per cent chance that it wouldn't work. That means, in non-mathematical language, it PROBABLY wouldn't work. Throw in a disastrous fertilisation day and subsequently weakened embryos and the chances were even more slight.

And yet, that morning when Rosie trembled in the bathroom, that little plastic stick was, to her, still the greatest chance she'd ever had of actually being a mother.

As she lay next to me after the stick had delivered its verdict, she shivered and cried and quite genuinely wanted the proverbial earth to open and swallow her, to end this pain and hide her predicament from others.

She was childless, barren, unfruitful, infecund. She was also getting old, her eggs were dying and all hope was dying with them. Even IVF didn't work. And she knew at some point in the coming hours she would have to tell people.

Spreading the bad news

However hard they try, people are generally shit at making you feel better if they've never been through what you've experienced.

Quite simply, like most things in life, unless you have done IVF you have absolutely no idea what it's like.

And that was the self-constructed brick wall Rosie had to tackle that morning.

First parents, then friends, then eventually everyone else to whom she happened to have mentioned that she was doing IVF. The list was long, painful and regrettable.

Which is why I repeat that top tip, right from the beginning: limit the number of people you tell that you are doing IVF. It just makes it all easier. Not because IVF is anything to be ashamed of – in fact the more we shout about it the more it might break the taboo that bizarrely still exists. No, limit the number of people you tell simply because in our experience it's one way of protecting her emotions through this pretty delicate period.

The madness begins again

I also knew that after these shitty few days and weeks the madness would begin again – and it would be even worse than ever.

I knew Rosie would want to do IVF again. Immediately. Or sooner.

And I knew that I didn't.

The day in the booth had genuinely scarred me and I wanted as little to do with fertility clinics as I possibly could.

It had also brought home the reality of the casino of life: the house always wins.

I also knew that if (= when) we did IVF again we would have to pay. We'd played our only NHS card and next time we would be looking at a bill of about seven grand.

But we were now on the IVF helter skelter, where you go round and round, trying and trying again, getting steadily older, poorer, and more desperate until we skidded on the ground on our backsides.

It's everything I feared about IVF from the beginning, as I'd heard too many stories.

Like a man I know who I shall call Pete who told me that he and his wife had done IVF five times, 'And we're about to try a sixth time,' he said with the helpless expression of a man who's been a half of the desperate whole. 'We're nearly broke and there's nothing I can do to talk her out of it.'

Goodbye, logic

The negative result confirmed the total lack of logic associated with IVF.

Yes, we know that the more you want something the less chance you have of getting it, but this is something you are told probably won't work and, hey, it doesn't.

So you try again and again and again, even though you know you're getting a little older and more desperate each time – both the enemies of successful fertilisation.

I also worried about all those IVF drugs.

These are powerful drugs that alter the workings of women's insides. It simply can't be good for you to take a drug to make you produce ten eggs or more. It just can't. Particularly if you take them several times. I feared, probably irrationally, an IVF time-bomb in about 30 years when they discover the actual long-term effects of fertility treatment.

The joy of perspective

But now, writing this, I realise how silly and trivial all of it is.

Because the second time we did IVF Rosie's pregnancy stick said 'yes'. The embryo didn't survive beyond eight weeks, but at least she'd made progress.

And the third time, the stick said 'yes' again and now there's a boisterous, squirmy, kicking thing in Rosie's stomach at the time of writing, so what the hell was I so worried about?

I say all this to hopefully give perspective.

When the time comes, if her pregnancy wee stick stays obstinately blank the world can seem the same way.

So please be aware of this, but hopefully you'll go into the whole thing better briefed and better equipped than we were and there will be no second or third or sixth time for you.

Oh, one final thing to also make me look like a negative old wanker;

I got an email a couple months ago from that man called Pete I mentioned earlier.

I told him that Rosie and I were doing a book about IVF to try to pass on what we'd learnt and save people a huge amount of the shit we'd been through, as I knew he'd been through even more than we had.

'Great idea' he emailed back. 'Wish we'd done a book, particularly as my wife is now four months pregnant. Can't believe it. That sixth go at IVF actually fucking worked.'

How to survive this stage

* Be aware that if it doesn't work, it's only in line with probability. The odds are it won't work. But don't say this out loud. Ever.

* Instead, try to gently discuss the possible outcomes BEFORE you start IVF and be aware that it might, just might, not work and what you would do if that were to possibly occur.

* Basically, try to come up with a survival plan even though neither of you will want to. By the time you start IVF this will be too late as positive thinking is EVERYTHING.

* And if – if – she does have a negative result, delve deep into your nice parts and cuddle and cosset the living shit out of her. You are her only ally at this stage and you can only imagine what pain she is going through.

The consultant says...

I think the most important thing is not to have any knee-jerk reactions if the outcome is negative.

It's important that you contact the specialist, plan a follow-up appointment and don't make any immediate decisions at this stage.

But certainly get that follow-up appointment, because the sooner you get the information you need to help you make decisions, the better.

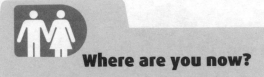

Where are you now?

You have had a negative result; IVF hasn't worked

*

You've cried a lot

*

You have told all the people you needed to tell

*

You have agreed with your partner if and when to try IVF again

*

You have researched the options for your next attempt

*

You have a plan of action

13

How to cope with a positive result

HER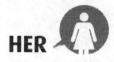

How to cope with a positive result

I know what you're thinking: 'What? How to cope? I don't need a chapter on how to cope. I'm overjoyed and that's it.'

And you're right, of course.

It's a milestone and an incredible relief but for me it was also a lesson that I had reached an amazing new stage but not quite the end of the process.

As I discovered, things don't always go to plan...

What happened to us

That second time we did IVF, it took me an unfeasibly long time to actually believe there were two lines on the test stick.

I held it up to the light, held it against a white wall, took it to the window, heart thumping away all the while with me wondering if this was finally it, if I had finally managed to get my first ever positive pregnancy test.

Eventually I took the test upstairs and woke Richard up to show him.

I needed clarification and I needed it now. He stumbled to the window to inspect my wee-stained test strip and pronounced that he could also see a second faint pink line.

I think then I finally let myself believe it.

We laughed and hugged and I shouted, 'I'm pregggggnaaaaant' in Slade fashion. Then we went back to bed and talked about what this all meant and the significance of those two little pink lines.

Start spreading the news

There were people to be told and it was so nice to phone my parents with good news for once – they had been through it all with us every step of the way and were just as anxious about the test day.

It was lovely to be able to tell my friends and brother as well. They were all delighted for me and it all felt quite euphoric and exciting.

It was also great to be able to phone the clinic and let them know the good news. They scheduled me in for a blood test the following day just to confirm the levels of HCG were good and a scan in three weeks to check for a heartbeat. A heartbeat!!

I also began experiencing symptoms the moment I declared myself officially pregnant. Of course I did.

I felt immediately nauseous and my boobs were sore. Nothing to do with the progesterone suppositories I was still taking, of course, oh no, these were now (in my head at least) bona fide pregnancy symptoms. I'm surprised I didn't immediately throw up into the nearest plastic bag.

Reality check

Once the elation of the result and first few hours subsided, the worry and waiting began again.

Because, when you've been through infertility and IVF you don't just assume a positive pregnancy test equals a baby. No, you know far too much about the whole process and words such as 'empty sac', 'blighted ovum' and 'ectopic pregnancy' loom large in your imagination.

And so back to Dr Google you go, checking out the symptoms for each

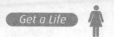

disaster scenario and wondering if that's what is going on inside your newly changed uterus.

More waiting

And of course you're back to the waiting.

You thought the two-week wait was bad, now try a three-week wait before your first 'viability' scan where they check to see if there really is a little live embryo splashing about in there.

They don't like to scan you before then as often a heartbeat can't be seen until after you are seven weeks' pregnant. So, you are back to practising being patient again. But it's a little different this time because although I was riddled with worry I tried to enjoy being PUPO (Pregnant Until Proven Otherwise).

Being pregnant for the first time

It was certainly fun walking around actually being pregnant for once.

I loved going to the supermarket and thinking, 'not sure I can have provolone cheese on my pizza, I'd better look that up.' Or abstaining from alcohol not because I was 'coming down with something' but because of my own secret reason. And going to sleep at night it was lovely to think about this little miracle of life growing inside me.

I did try hard not to get too far ahead of myself, though. I knew it was a long, long road until I would actually hold a baby in my arms so I tried to pace myself mentally. Not easy to do when you've got a great big carrot being dangled in front of you that can potentially make all your dreams come true.

But I also knew how quickly it could all be snatched away. I absolutely hoped and believed that it was going to be okay but I couldn't rely on it, I knew that much.

Still, we approached that seven-week scan with a fair amount of positivity and hopefulness.

I was feeling some actual symptoms – a bit sick, bloated and boob tenderness – and generally felt like there was definitely something going on in there.

The first scan

And so back to the clinic, legs open wide and there on the screen was the confirmation I'd always wanted.

A little growing embryo with a flickering heartbeat that you could see, but not yet hear.

It was amazing to see this little pulsing light showing us that it had worked and I was definitely properly pregnant.

A sense of triumph washed over me – we had finally done it.

For the first time in my 36 years on the planet, I was actually growing another human inside me. And all thanks to the wonderful team at my clever clinic, oh yes, and Richard of course. Brilliant.

The happiness bubble was to last a little bit longer, but sadly not forever.

Tell-tale signs?

Looking back, perhaps there was a clue in the fact that the embryo was measuring just slightly smaller than it should (about the size it should be at six weeks, five days instead of seven weeks), but still within normal range.

Or perhaps lovely Liz the sonographer had an inkling that our little heartbeat didn't sound too strong. Perhaps it was her long experience that prompted her to advise we come back for a ten-week progress scan with them rather than just skipping straight ahead to the 12-week NHS scan. 'Just in case...' she said.

But at the time there was no indication that anything was up, and we skipped out of the clinic, blurry scan photo in hand, delighted with ourselves and our tiny pulsating embryo.

We'd done it!

I'd properly got pregnant!

Whether I would stay pregnant, of course, was another matter entirely...

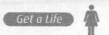

Your baby in fruit and veg

4 weeks pregnant = the size of a poppy seed	The cells of the placenta are growing in the lining of your uterus. It will soon be able to make nutrients for your baby and remove waste products.
7 weeks pregnant = the size of a pea	Fingers and toes are becoming distinct and the baby is moving in fits and starts.
10 weeks pregnant = the size of a kidney bean	No longer an embryo, it is now officially a fetus weighing just under 4g. It's increasingly active, swallowing fluid and kicking its new limbs.
12 weeks pregnant = the size of a large plum	Your baby can now close its fingers and curl its toes. And its reflexes are developing. If you prod your belly it will move, although you probably can't feel it yet.

increasing odds, week by week

If the early scan picks up a heartbeat on the baby, research has shown that if you then see a heartbeat at:

- 6 weeks of pregnancy, the chances of the pregnancy continuing are 78%

- 8 weeks, the chances of the pregnancy continuing are 98%

- 10 weeks, the chances of the pregnancy continuing are 99.4%

How to survive this stage

* If you can't believe it, do a few different pregnancy tests to confirm – the last thing you want is to get excited and then find out it was just your eyes deceiving you.

* Tell people but don't tell everyone. It's lovely to finally share some good news with your close friends and family who have been willing this to happen for you BUT don't tell everyone you meet, it just makes it harder if the worst happens.

* Remember you've got a long way to go. You're at four weeks out of a possible 40. You're only a tenth of the way there. You need to pace yourself and your expectations of what's to come.

* But celebrate. For God's sake celebrate. You've been through enough crap that you should grasp at these positive moments. Go out together and enjoy your good news.

* Behave as if you're pregnant. You may as well start eating well and taking care of yourself now and assume this is all going to work out.

* Stay off Google if you can. Yes, you know there are many things that can go wrong now but really, what's the point in stressing about them? I know I didn't really manage this but I really wish I had.

* Try not to think about pregnancy 24/7. Find ways to distract your thoughts – work, films, whatever it takes. Give yourself an hour a day to think about it, but other than that, pretend you're completely 'normal'.

* Don't buy any baby books, or any baby things – not yet.

* Try not to invent or over-analyse your symptoms. Yes, it could be the pregnancy hormones kicking in, but equally it could also be the progesterone, which (very helpfully) gives you all the symptoms of pregnancy.

HIM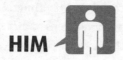

How to cope with a positive result

This should all be piss, quite literally.

Her wee-wee pregnancy stick has shown up positive, so that's it, isn't it? Job done.

Well, nearly, yes.

Just a couple of lessons we learnt about celebrating too soon...

What happened to us

So shocking was the appearance of a faint pink line on Rosie's pregnancy stick during our second IVF attempt that she kept repositioning herself around the room for different points of light.

It *looked* like there was a line but maybe she could see it just because she wanted so much to see one.

It had been a five-year build-up to all this.

She'd already been through one failed cycle and had never been pregnant at all, ever, during her entire life so maybe this was just a trick of the light? That is, the light coming from all the 17 different vantage points she'd chosen to hold it up and stare at it.

My first feeling was one of shock at how badly I wanted there to be a little pinky red line.

I say 'shock' because my original position when I first met Rosie eight years earlier was NOT WANTING CHILDREN AT ALL UNDER ANY CIRCUMSTANCES EVER. The idea was abhorrent.

From what I'd read and heard from primary sources and actual owners of the things, babies had a strong tradition of growing into children.

Yes, children.

Greedy, snotty, stinky, shouty, self-centred pieces of ungovernable scum who wake you up early, make you feel guilty, scream about nothing, ruin your holidays, draw on your walls and wee on your gardens, drain you of all resources, lie to you and tell you how much they hate you, and then eventually leave your home, having reduced you to lined, greying pieces of rubble, to spend their adult lives meticulously but steadily reducing the amount of time they ever have to spend with you.

And yet from that original position I am now standing in our bedroom urging there to be a pink line on my wife's pregnancy test.

I haven't gone to the other extreme, of course – I still don't desperately want children – but I don't vehemently not want them either and, above all else, I just can't bear the idea of Rosie never having any.

As she repositioned the little plastic stick to another vantage point, my invaluable expertise, well, mostly the fact that I own a pair of eyes, was called in for final confirmation.

Yup. It was as faint as a deep-vein thrombosis but there did look to be a line.

Finally.

The woman who, about seven years earlier and just four weeks into our drunk, gropey, fledgling relationship, had warned me that she would want children eventually (a little creepy, perhaps, a little too soon? Oh, okay, well I suppose at least you're being honest) was finally going to have one.

Telling the world

Three hours later everyone she knew was also aware of this. I mean, everyone.

Family, friends, friends of friends, cousins of friends of friends, the postman, local newsagent, people on their way to work, old people in parks, all the staff at Waitrose, next door's cat, the various cat friends of next door's cat.

For several hours all I could hear upstairs was Rosie repeatedly shouting into her phone 'It's fucking worked!!! I'm pregnant!!!!!!!!'

My instinctive reaction, uncharacteristically portentous, was caution. I've heard stuff about something called 'the 12-week scan' and that women don't normally tell people they're pregnant until then because that's the stage when they're less likely to miscarry or something.

I didn't really want people to know... you know, just in case. But at that stage it really wasn't about me. It was about Rosie.

A positive test is about uncontrollable delight and relief and a woman who wants the world to know that she is normal. And that she can at last mix with women with babies and join in their conversations about babies and talk about being fat and pregnant.

Finally she'd won and we'd reached the end of this absurd, draining process.

Our only mistake – mine included – was that we hadn't factored in reality; in particular that cruel mother, nature.

We knew the whole thing about not telling anyone you're pregnant until 12 weeks. Even I'd heard that. But the relief made us feel slightly invincible. We'd finally bloody done it and that was that.

In natural, non-assisted conception, at this stage this would all be irrelevant. Most women barely know they're pregnant that early on and so just carry on as normal, non-assisted women.

The normal first scan isn't until 12 weeks. With IVF, of course, things are rather different. Every single detail and stage has been monitored and every bit of you has been scanned and prodded so it's only natural that they will check on progress earlier too.

The first scan

And so there's more waiting.

We know everything will be okay, but there's a wait until the first scan confirms everything.

And so, three weeks later we go for the first scan.

A little trepidation, of course, but there it is.

The ultrasound lady goes up Rosie's insides with her magic vaginal probe and there, on the TV screen, is a little pulsating bean.

It's a heartbeat. An actual heartbeat. Of a baby growing inside Rosie's womb.

She cries with barely contained elation. It really has worked.

Perhaps we should have picked up on signals, like the cautious but kind way that Liz, the ultrasound lady, said to celebrate this moment but to be aware there was a 'long way to go and sometimes it's wise to have another scan in a couple of weeks rather than waiting until that landmark 12-week moment'.

And a couple of weeks later we see Liz again and with a gentle professionalism and sensitivity we were lucky to have, Liz softly points out that there is no longer a heartbeat and the little pulsating bean has gone.

More on how to cope with that landfill of life shit in the next chapter.

But it was yet another IVF lesson: the odds are on your side when you see the heartbeat but, contrary to what all those morons said to Rosie about it being 'the best sign and that definitely means you'll have a healthy baby', the odds of survival are greatly improved after 12 weeks.

And that, of course, is why, in natural conception, they do the scan then and not before.

Know your dates

Everything in pregnancy is measured in weeks. These are the key times you should know about if you wish to show her how interested and engaged you are with her insides. Also, you'll probably get dragged along to these events anyway, so they're worth knowing about in advance.

4 weeks	That's how pregnant she is at the time of the positive test. The mother of something the size of a pin-head
7 weeks	This will be when you do your first scan (only for IVF treatment – usually it's at 12 weeks)
10 weeks	Sometimes she'll have a progress scan now just to make sure everything's okay (again usually only for IVF-ers)

12 weeks	You're back in the NHS. This is the first scan for all new mums. They check the baby looks okay, take lots of measurements, confirm it's in the right place and has the right number of bits. This is the truly weird one as you try to muster up some paternal love for what looks like a squirming, translucent alien.
16 weeks	She might want to have a private scan about now as it's the first time they can really tell you the sex of the baby. I still don't understand why some people don't want to know this. 'We wanted it to be a surprise' is what they always say. Why? It just means that if you wanted a boy you'll be disappointed and vice versa. Knowing we had a daughter meant I could start my preparation for all the arguments, lies and twat-awful boyfriends in about 15 years' time.
20 weeks	Another routine NHS scan where they take all sorts of other measurements and can confirm the sex if you want to know. Don't be disappointed if it looks like your unborn son has inherited SOME DISTANT RELATIVE'S tiny penis. It might just be because the baby is actually a girl.
26–30 weeks	The time you can get one of those stupid and absurd '4D' scans where you'll pay a large amount of money for a photo of what looks like a fistful of butter and mud fashioned into the vague shape of a mashed human.
40 weeks-ish	Chances are you won't see your baby again until they're born. They are due 40 weeks from day one. Actually, they come whenever they want to, anything before 37 weeks is classed as premature, anything over 42 weeks (294 days) is overdue and generally after 42 weeks they'll want to prise it out with a shoehorn and a hoover or something.

Learning from mistakes... yet again

So... the third time we did IVF, we knew what we were doing.

The wee-wee stick came up lined, Rosie was overjoyed but, because she'd only told a handful of people that she was doing IVF, there was only an even smaller handful of people to tell that she was pregnant and that it was only early stages but for now she was happy.

And when we saw the little pulsating bean again at seven weeks we were relieved but cautious. It was another stage, but we'd been here before.

But at ten weeks when it was still there, well, to be fair Rosie did go a little mental with joy then. And at 12 weeks she could finally behave like a woman who was pregnant.

This time it actually had worked. We'd made it.

I just wish, with the human mind's wonderful gift for retrospect, we had known all this that very first time we did IVF.

How to survive this stage

* She won't want to hear about the possibility of the pregnancy not resulting in an actual baby, so again, if you can, gently talk about all this stuff before you start IVF. It's as hard as hell to be heard in all the madness, but just try. Temper your delight. Curb your enthusiasm.

* As I've said before, try to limit the number of people you tell – it makes it so much easier if it doesn't work out as planned.

* The 12-week pregnancy scan is there for a reason – we know that now. Celebrate each stage but remember that nature is a clever beast and only lets the healthiest survive.

* Thank all your gods that you are a man because it must be hideous to have all this baby-making stuff to contend with.

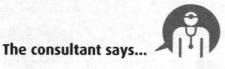

The consultant says...

A positive test is great news but it is only a start as a proportion of people who get pregnant will miscarry.

Once you get beyond the six-week scan, and then the eight-week scan, the more your chances of success increase.

It's why the 12-week scan is so important because only a very small percentage of women will miscarry after 12 weeks.

Where are you now?

You have had a positive pregnancy test, possibly for the first time ever

*

You have celebrated and told your nearest and dearest

*

The worry might have started to set in

*

You have been back for one or two early scans

*

You are holding your breath until that 12-week scan

14

Diary of a miscarriage

HER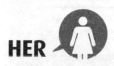

Diary of a miscarriage

Hopefully you won't need to read this chapter. It's just here in case.

But if it does happen to you I thought it might be useful to explain what I went through, to reassure you that you are certainly not alone and that you will come out the other side of the experience absolutely fine.

It felt particularly hard after IVF as, after seeing a heartbeat on the seven-week scan, I felt like I'd finally made it.

This was yet another lesson to learn the hard way.

What happened to us

A common experience

I didn't realise quite how common miscarriages were until I had one.

Then, of course, the sad secret came out from lots of friends and colleagues who had all been through it.

Everyone had different experiences; from some hardly knowing they were pregnant to others who faced the horror of actually giving birth to a stillborn baby.

Miscarriage facts

- It is estimated that approximately 20 per cent of all pregnancies miscarry, with the majority (up to 85 per cent) doing so in weeks 1 to 12.[1]

- 1 in 100 women will experience recurrent miscarriages (three or more successive miscarriages).[2]

- From a mental health point of view, up to a third of women attending specialist clinics as a result of miscarriage are clinically depressed.[3]

1 National Institute for Health and Care Excellence, Ectopic pregnancy and miscarriage, clinical guideline CG154, London NICE, 2012. Available at: guidance.nice.org.uk/CG154 (accessed 18 February 2014)
2 Royal College of Obstetricians and Gynaecologists, The effects of a miscarriage on future pregnancies, London RCOG, 2008. Available at: www.rcog.org.uk/news/effects-first-miscarriage-future-pregnancies (accessed 18 February 2014)
3 Rai R, Regan L, Recurrent miscarriage. Lancet 2006; 368(9535): 601–11

And everyone felt differently about it – some felt it was a clever twist of nature, sifting out unhealthy embryos, while others still felt the pain of loss quite acutely despite it being years ago and having had more children since.

We all feel these experiences differently and it's not a competition to see who has suffered the most and deserves the most sympathy.

For me, I took it pretty hard but strangely not quite as hard as the first failed IVF attempt.

By my reckoning I had at least been pregnant for a short while and so I felt that this was some sort of progress. I couldn't bear the idea of going through the IVF process from scratch again and there's no doubt that throwing IVF into the mix does give miscarriage an extra sting in its tail, but I knew I wasn't defeated by it yet. Even at the height of my grief I knew I was prepared to do it all again.

It's strange to describe it as grief because, arguably, it's not really a proper living creature at that early stage.

However, it felt like I'd lost something real, at least in terms of my hopes, dreams and finally some good fortune coming my way. But life goes on and time is a great healer – and other trite clichés that people tell

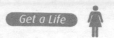

you so often that you want to punch them in the face, but they turn out to be true in the end.

So, here is how it happened for me, again with the caveat that I know many, many women have had it worse and tragically, more than once. This is just my version in all its gory detail.

The timeline

Just to give you a sense of timescale for my second round of IVF:

- **2 March 2012: I started the first set of IVF drugs**

- **27 March 2012: Egg collection**

- **30 March 2012: Embryo transfer**

- **11 April 2012: I did my pregnancy test** at home and for the first time EVER saw a positive result: that elusive double line.
  I was completely overjoyed and remember waking Richard up by shouting a war cry of 'I'm preg….nant!!'.

  I cautiously told my nearest and dearest then held my breath until the first scan back at the clinic on 7 May, when I was officially around seven weeks' pregnant.

- **7 May 2012: the first scan**
  I can't quite explain the joy of seeing that little light pulsing away inside a grey blob on the screen. It was a heartbeat and it was ours.

  The print-out of the scan photo given to us by Liz the sonographer was put up on the fridge and I said hello to it every day. It didn't look like anything at all, really, perhaps a wonky kidney bean, certainly nothing resembling a baby, but my friends and family dutifully cooed over it when they came to visit.

  It may have looked like a little grey smudge, but they knew it was a big deal to us.

  We started to call it Eric the Bee. I don't know why. I think because it was spring and there were a lot of bees around and we thought it was funny.

It was nice sitting there in the evening thinking about our little bee growing inside me. I felt a bit sick and bloated, had sore boobs and began to believe that the dark times had lifted and we had finally got lucky.

• 23 May: the 10-week scan

Then on 23 May we went for our ten-week scan back with the same sonographer and had the carpet pulled out from under us.

Again, Liz was quick and as soon as that ultrasound probe went in, she looked at the screen, made a heartfelt noise in the back of her throat which I shall never forget and said 'I'm really sorry, I've got bad news.'

I was so completely in disbelief I fully expected her to then crack a smile and say, 'Only joking!', and we would all roll around laughing.

But I quickly realised she would not be allowed to do that and that she must be telling the truth.

I looked to Richard for help.

I really didn't know what I was supposed to feel or how to react.

I just had to listen to her kind words and try to process what she was saying.

Richard, of course, wanted to know some facts and get an explanation, so Liz showed him the small, feeble shape on the screen and how much bigger she would have expected it to measure at this stage and where the heartbeat should have been.

They talked about embryo growth and chromosomes and possible reasons why this had happened and I just lay there staring at the screen, willing it to start pulsating again just as we had seen it do only a few weeks before.

All the while I lay there with this probe up my vagina and clasping Richard's sweaty hand, feeling very vulnerable, with my heart sinking as she took the probe out. And that was it, that was the end of our baby.

No warning

Liz explained that we'd had a 'missed miscarriage', in that there were no signs of miscarriage, no cramping or bleeding, the embryo had just stopped developing. The embryo was actually measuring smaller than it had been at the previous scan so the heartbeat had probably stopped soon after we saw it.

The gestational sac that housed the embryo had, however, continued to grow (and, in a cruel twist, give off pregnancy symptoms) so even though there was no pregnancy I still felt sick, had sore boobs and was bloated, etc.

The shock

It's funny what comes into your head at moments like these. I just kept thinking, 'Oh God, I've got to tell everyone'.

It's a strange feeling of shock with no real tears yet. Just an empty feeling of not believing it's real.

I remember feeling like this before at strangely dramatic moments (like splitting up with boyfriends) where it feels like you're watching yourself in a film and wanting to act out your reactions in a way you've seen other people do. I gave Richard a hug and tried a sort of strange crying but it didn't come naturally... yet.

Just another miscarriage...

Lovely Liz, who was practical, upbeat and still very sympathetic, arranged for us to see one of the consultants in her office.

We sat down and the consultant breezed in and we shook hands and smiled dutifully in the polite English way.

She gave us the facts and stats about miscarriage and the likely cause being problems with the genetic development (none of which we could really take in) and then told us what was going to happen next. We were told we had to make a decision about letting it all happen naturally or having a procedure called an ERPC (evacuation of remaining products of conception).

She told us the operation could cause scarring in the uterus and that although unlikely she knew of one woman who had scarring so bad she was forced to use a surrogate.

She also said that waiting to miscarry naturally could be a long painful process that could also lead to complications if it didn't all come out of it's own accord and then you have to have an ERPC anyway. Great.

She wrote a letter for our GP and gave us lots of bits of paper. Meanwhile we were about 17 steps behind her and wanted to know why and how did 'missed miscarriage' happen, when did it happen?

Why was the embryo smaller than when we first saw it?

She told us that when the embryo dies it hangs down its head and starts to curl up and shrink. Richard later told me how sad this made him feel. It was the first time the consultant had talked about the embryo in terms that sounded anything vaguely human and it hit us both hard to think of this tiny little thing giving up on life and shrivelling up to die.

After a few more questions the consultant was clearly needed elsewhere.

She took a phone call and we heard her say, just within earshot, 'I can't, I'm dealing with a miscarriage'. The comment hurt but it was then that I realised how common miscarriages really are and how the clinic had to deliver this news to people several times every day.

She got up to show us out of the room and we complied, feeling scared, confused and utterly bewildered when only an hour we had walked into the clinic feeling excited and happy.

Outside the clinic

We left the clinic and as soon as we got outside we both started crying.

This time it was for real. We are not used to crying on the street but we couldn't help it.

We walked around the corner and, with immaculate British timing, bumped into our next-door neighbour.

It was lunchtime and he was running with a colleague. We managed to compose ourselves briefly.

'How funny bumping into you here,' he said. 'Have you been in there?'

He pointed. There is a big exhibition opposite the hospital. So big that we'd failed to even notice it.

'No' Richard said, We've just been in... er... there... having a miscarriage...'

The neighbour stared, a slightly unexpected end to his polite conversation and ran off with his colleague.

On the walk back to the train station we popped into Pret-A-Manger and I realised I could eat whatever I liked so I bought a ham and brie sandwich as if to spite my dead embryo. The journey home was surreal. We ate our sandwiches on the train and made crap jokes and talked about how, why, it could have happened.

We saw the embryo at seven weeks. We saw a heartbeat.

Back home

We called the two-and-a-half weeks that followed our 'grief holiday'.

It happened to coincide with an abnormally hot spring and, whilst everyone was making the most of the sunshine, we were lying around combining sunbathing with bouts of crying.

Fortunately I was having a break from work at the time so I was able to fully indulge my grief, which really helped get it all out of my system.

People came over to cheer me up and everyone sent lovely messages, and of course my parents were brilliant and kept popping over with cake and jokes and positive reassurances.

I just had the overwhelming urge to stay at home.

I couldn't bear to be out in public for fear of bumping into someone I knew and bursting into tears inappropriately. I even tried to limit trips to the supermarket.

I felt perfectly happy and safe at home and just wanted to stay put, preferably until I was heavily pregnant and could finally face everyone. Obviously that wasn't an option.

Wanting to be normal

The trouble was that every time I left the house I felt totally exposed. Now it wasn't just pregnant women or women with babies and kids that upset me but anyone walking down the street looking vaguely happy. I so wanted to be happy and carefree again. I wanted to be back to my normal self, before all this obsession and difficulty with having babies reared its ugly head.

I desperately wished I could persuade myself that I didn't even want a baby anymore, just so I could get on with my life. I never used to be a depressed person and I hated what I'd become. I'd put my life on hold for the past few years and all that I had to show for it was a fading positive pregnancy test in a drawer. I missed my old, happy life. I missed me.

Some time during this embarrassing period of self-pity came, I believe, a turning point.

I was so sick of being an 'infertile' and all the misery that came with it that I started to actually contemplate a life without children. I certainly wasn't okay with it and hoped it wasn't my future, but I did start to at least contemplate it.

For the first time ever.

In a way it was quite liberating. I thought about what Richard and I could do with all that spare time and money and it wasn't all that bad. It at least made me think that if the worst happened and we were never successful then at least I would cope. I wouldn't shrivel up and die like our little bean and I wouldn't hide inside like I had been doing the past few weeks. Somehow we would actually be okay. I basically decided at that point that whatever happened I would not let childlessness and loss define my life. I would bloody well live it, no matter what.

The actual miscarriage

Emotionally, this was progress, of course, but physically I was way behind and still had not had an actual miscarriage. I was walking around with this dead embryo inside me and it was starting to freak me out a little.

I had decided against getting the ERPC operation and wanted to let things happen naturally. The consultants said they were prepared to give it a few weeks and if nothing had happened after three weeks they would urge me to have the op.

So, I waited and waited and read endless 'miscarriage diaries' on the internet.

I was ready to bleed and let it all go. And finally, two-and-a-half weeks after our devastating scan, and probably four-and-a-half weeks after the embryo died, it began.

I had a little bit of bleeding for a few days, gradually getting heavier, and then on Sunday 10 June I woke up to proper period cramps.

But they were different to normal; they would come on and then stop, rather than be the constant ache that always came with my period. They kept coming, in spurts and increasing in intensity, but still giving me a bit of respite in between.

I realise now that these mirrored (in some small way) contraction pains and it was a strangely familiar (yet different) sort of pain.

The bleeding got heavier and I was soaking a pad with blood every few hours (no tampons allowed) and I kept going to the toilet and passing large clots. Then, at about lunchtime, I felt a really big pain and an urge to go to the loo and felt something solid pass out of my vagina.

It was a really weird feeling, unlike anything I'd felt before, a bit like my insides were falling out, and I remember feeling quite scared and calling Richard for reassurance. But I knew really what had happened.

The sac and embryo had passed.

I did look into the toilet but it was just a sea of red blood and I think that was probably a good thing. I never saw what remained of the little flashing heartbeat we'd named Eric the Bee. It was gone and I was grateful that it had all happened quite quickly and relatively painlessly.

The recovery

The residual bleeding eased off after about a week and I had to keep going back to the clinic for scans to check the womb lining had all come away, but after a few more weeks I began to feel a bit more normal.

I actually felt quite good that my body had done what it needed to do and I felt a bit more in tune with my natural processes, more than I had in the few years I'd been trying and failing to conceive.

I did, however, think that it was ridiculous that my body could miscarry successfully, yet not actually conceive successfully.

But nevertheless I was back to normal, with no lasting scars (except the emotional ones) and felt ready to give my body a break and get a bit of me back that wasn't obsessed with follicles and eggs and embryos and genetic disorders.

We had a follow-up consultation on 11 July back at the clinic (four and a half months after I'd started the drugs) where I was told it was just one of those things, very common and there was no reason not to try again.

And we knew already that we would. In a stroke of good fortune, we'd moved house and discovered that we could get another round of IVF on the NHS. We were lucky, and despite all the trauma we were so grateful that we could give it another go.

But at that point we were ready for a break. And perhaps most importantly we were ready to welcome a bit of joy into our lives that didn't start and end with having a baby.

Yes, it was time to get a dog.

Types of miscarriage

- **Threatened miscarriage**
  This is when you have bleeding early in your pregnancy and your cervix (the opening to your uterus) is tightly closed. In about half of all women who have a threatened miscarriage the pregnancy continues successfully.

- **Inevitable miscarriage**
  Usually just called a miscarriage. This is when you have bleeding early in your pregnancy and your cervix is open, which means your pregnancy will be lost.

- **Incomplete miscarriage**
  This is when you have had a miscarriage but there is still some tissue left in your uterus.

- **Complete miscarriage**
  This means that you have lost your pregnancy and your uterus is empty.

- **Delayed, missed or silent miscarriage**
  This means that although your developing baby has died, you haven't had any bleeding or lost any tissue.

Source: www.bupa.co.uk/individuals/health-information/directory/m/miscarriage

How to survive a miscarriage

- Talk to other women who've had one. Their empathy and understanding will be soothing – it really is – and hopefully they will have proved that time does heal.

- Take time to grieve. There is no shortcut here; embrace the sadness, however badly it hits you. Better to address it now than for it to rear its ugly unfinished head in years to come.

- Seek professional help if you are really suffering. There's only so much your friends and family can say. Your clinic will offer counselling and it's a good opportunity for you both as a couple to discuss your feelings.

- Whether you are miscarrying at home or in hospital, if you have the chance, be prepared and don't do it alone. Have your husband/friend/mum with you and stock up on painkillers, big pads, hot-water bottles and chocolate.

- Don't feel bad about keeping scan pictures, test sticks or any other mementos from your pregnancy experience. You were attached to that little bean and there's no need to destroy your memories until you're completely ready to let go.

- Having said that, try to find some way of saying goodbye. A lovely neighbour gave me a little rose bush to plant and I felt like that was my gesture towards closure.

- Keep talking to your partner about it but don't be surprised or angry if they seem to be moving on faster than you.

- Give your body a break, it's been through a lot. Take some time off IVF or even trying to get pregnant for at least a month and do whatever feels like healing – yoga, massage, hot baths, exercise.

- Book a holiday. Particularly a holiday that you couldn't go on if you were pregnant/had kids. We opted for a posh spa hotel.

- Get a dog (or another significant distraction). If it wasn't for our miscarriage we would never have got Jeremy (yes, he really is called that – it's a long story...) and now we can't imagine life without him.

HIM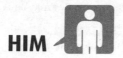

Diary of a miscarriage

You don't need to read this chapter and hopefully you won't have any reason to; it's just here in case.

Mostly because we weren't prepared for it.

We hadn't even thought about it. Why would we?

Miscarriages were things that happened to mums and sisters and other people.

Stupid thinking, really, given how common they are.

But because we didn't know anything about them we didn't know what to expect and had no idea about the strain it would put on us.

So this is what we went through, how we dealt with it and hopefully it will be useful if you find yourself in a similar position.

What happened to us

I'd heard of miscarriages, of course, but we didn't really know what they were.

I tended to think of them in the context of Justice – or rather, injustice – and men in denim from the 1970s, often in small groups that sounded like *Blake's 7*, being wrongfully imprisoned by over-zealous or vote-hungry home secretaries.

In the context of human life – or rather, death – I knew people who'd had them.

Loads of people.

And loads of miscarriages.

I think my sister had two of them. I think my mother also had two. I think. I don't know because it seemed so far away in time and place.

Not that I didn't think they were awful. They were. Probably. I didn't know because I'd never actually asked anyone about them. Or maybe I did. And maybe they didn't want to talk about it.

At no time during our increasingly desperate efforts to make a baby – first naturally and then using drugs and pots – did we ever really discuss it. Not because we were deliberately blocking it out, like many of the nastier elements of IVF, just because we genuinely didn't factor it in. Utterly idiotic given what we know now.

If miscarriages happened, they probably happened later in pregnancy or something – and always to other people.

After the patience-testing two-week wait, even the joy of the positive urine stick is nothing compared to that first scan at seven weeks. There on the screen is a little pulsating thing, like an overweight cursor.

'That's its heartbeat' said Liz the sonographer, who I always preferred to call 'the ultrasound lady'.

Its heartbeat. Our baby's heartbeat. Our baby's actual heartbeat at seven weeks of age.

My first thought, shortly after the miracle of life, etc., etc., is what an amazing bit of kit a heart is.

You mean that little pump inside that bean will keep going until it is finally felled by fags or booze or stress or disease or old age? That means, bad genes and bad habits to one side it might keep pumping like that for another 80 years? Never even a day off or a holiday? Remarkable.

And there it was at the start of its thumping, throbbing ventricular life, its long pumpy road ahead. And we created it.

Finally.

We'd actually done it.

As Rosie got dressed, Liz encouraged measured celebration, pointing out that it was a milestone 'but there's still a long way to go'.

We nodded, knowing we would ignore her.

She suggested coming back for a check up at the ten-week mark, about three weeks from then, rather than waiting another five weeks for the standard 12-week scan. We agreed and thought nothing more of it.

Eric the Bee

Our bean was, for some reason neither of us knew, given the name Eric the Bee. Possibly because it was a warm late spring and there were bees all over the apple blossom. Or because it was actually nearly the size of a bee. Or because bees are nice. Or because of that Python song, even though the Eric in that case is just a 'demi-bee'.

There was delirium and delight in our house at last. The four-year shit-awful journey of drugs and probes and humiliation, pain and despair was finally at an end. Rosie was pregnant like any other pregnant woman, the pressure was off her (and me) and we could pick up where we left off.

'I'm afraid it's gone'

I even took the piss out of her absurd worrying on the way into the clinic three weeks later.

'What if it's not there?' Rosie kept saying.

'Of course it's there. Where's it gone? If it wasn't there, you wouldn't feel swollen and sick and pregnant. Besides, hearts like Eric's don't suddenly just stop.'

As I predicted, Rosie was shaking as she de-trousered and climbed on to the bed in Liz the ultrasound lady's room.

She reached for my hand. She was clammy and shaky. Yuck. I held on, doing my husband bit even though she was clearly making a silly fuss.

Liz didn't use the squirty-hair-gel-on-stomach route – it's still apparently too early for that – so it was just up Rosie's front entrance as usual with one of those special cameras on a stick.

We followed progress on the screen as she tried to find our Eric.

She told us to be patient as it was only small and sometimes hard to find.

The pause turned into an interlude. Almost a gap. Just blackness on the screen. Finally the clammy silence was broken.

'Oh dear, Rosie,' said Liz the ultrasound lady. 'I'm so sorry. I've got bad news. I'm afraid it's gone.'

Total silence. Rosie's hands shook even more.

Rosie couldn't seem to speak.

'Er... not there?' I said, in tones so high they could have attracted local dogs.

Liz explained that it had probably been dead a week or more as it was noticeably smaller than it had been at our seven-week scan.

Rosie still couldn't speak and just stared at me. There was no blood in her face, she couldn't blink and looked like someone whose soul had been mugged.

Eventually she slid off the bed and tried to get dressed. She couldn't seem to control her legs.

The missing piece of the jigsaw

Between us we tried to find out what might have happened and Liz explained it like a jigsaw puzzle.

The embryo requires all the right bits of DNA from Rosie and I to click together, she told our tattered faces, and if one or more of the pieces is missing, nature steps in.

'This isn't a baby that should have survived and I'm afraid it's nature making life easier for you. It knew this isn't a baby that was right.'

As someone who probably has to tell people a similar thing many times each week of her working life, with that succinct combination of science and sensitivity, Liz the ultrasound lady was a master of diplomacy, kindness, straight-talking, warmth and empathy.

Just another miscarriage

Liz told us to wait in another room, not to rush, and in about half an hour we would see one of the specialists. It's what they do in these circumstances.

At some point, we went into an office and a woman explained that these things just happen, usually for no reason. She gave us some forms to sign and explained what would happen next.

The embryo and the womb lining should dislodge itself in the next few weeks. It would be a bloody experience and often quite painful. If it didn't discharge by three weeks Rosie would have a procedure to forcibly extract it to prevent infection. We nodded, tear-streaked, exhausted, shocked, barely taking any of it in.

But why did it die and how and when?

She explained the raw facts and we tried to understand. I think it was the line about it having 'curled up and just died' that pierced my armour.

And then I seemed to be crying and pretending that I wasn't. I had never thought that I cared about all this rubbish, but I clearly really did.

The phone rang.

The woman turned to answer it. She was clearly wanted at something.

'Yes, okay, I'll be there when I can,' she said quietly. 'I'm dealing with a miscarriage.'

Yes, we were shells of ourselves, mere shadows. Our souls had been trampled on and our invisible architecture dismantled. But ultimately that's what we were. Another miscarriage.

And there would probably be another one in these seats in just a moment.

It was a stark reminder that this was just a medical procedure and miscarriages are very much a part of procreation, a nasty fact of life that we needed to deal with.

The running man

We shuffled out of the building clutching forms.

We didn't say anything to each other. We were still crying.

Round the corner we saw two men running towards us.

'Hi there!' said one, absurdly keenly.

We nodded or stared.

He was sweaty and it was probably lunchtime and he was probably one of those twats who leaves his office on a warm day like this in early summer to run around with a fat colleague rather than just sitting in the sun and eating food.

'What are you up to?' he said, still jogging on the spot.

Oh God. We realised it was one of our neighbours. Could this moment really be any more British?

'What?' I said.

'What are you up to round here – have you been to the exhibition?'

He pointed. There was a huge marquee across the road hosting a vast exhibition that we had carefully managed not to notice when we arrived.

'No...' I said, quite unable to remember the rules of how to behave when bumping into someone you barely know in the middle of a personal crisis. 'We haven't....um... in there,' I gestured to the clinic. 'We've been in there.... having a miscarriage.'

There followed one of those pauses that Richard Curtis might attempt in one of his films but he could never do it as well as this.

'Oh, okay,' said the sweaty man who lived next door. 'See you around.'

And he ran away with his colleague and we walked to the train station silently trying to work out just what the hell we do about making a family now.

People to tell, always people to tell

There were people to tell.

As there always is with IVF.

Loads of them.

Because everyone knew we were doing this. And even more people knew that Rosie was pregnant.

But we didn't want to talk to anyone.

Rosie phoned people and friends and family were unreasonably nice, doing all they could to try to understand what Rosie was going through and mostly failing and turning into vicariously grieving clichés.

We spent the next few days just lying in the sun. Always good when a personal setback of this magnitude coincides with good weather.

Oh no. I actually care.

What surprised me most was what was happening to me.

I kept doing normal boring things like making a sandwich or shaving or doing a poo and then bursting into tears. I couldn't control it. It was the bee. Curling up and dying. I just couldn't handle it. It was pulling me to bits. Our little Eric and what he might have been.

I didn't tell Rosie because it wasn't helpful, but it was a personal revelation.

Having resolutely never ever wanted children and never having seen the point of them but eventually tried to have one because I couldn't bear the idea of my beautiful wife growing old and childless and, after all, because I'd agreed on week four of our relationship to have them just so I might be able to have a go on her breasts, it was a revelation that me – the me I've always thought I've known – ACTUALLY FUCKING CARED.

Until this point I'd always felt pretty detached from the reality of what we were doing – you know, the whole 'trying to make a baby' stuff – but now we had actually made one and for some reason we'd never know he had curled up and died and I would never meet him.

Things I'll never do

Even worse I couldn't help myself imagining all those stupid and unhelpful things I should have firewalled out of my imagination.

I kept thinking of all the films I would never see with him and the football we'd never play. And how I'd never teach him about conkers and planets and dinosaurs and Laurel and Hardy and all the music and places I love. And we'd never laugh together when we knew we shouldn't and I'd never sit in a pub or drive to the coast and spot the sea and never giggle over silly words for the male member and women's knockers.

I imagined a whole six years – in colour and 3D with a lilting piano backdrop – that I'd never actually see and I was in pieces.

The wait...

Luckily the next stage was something we knew a lot about and had become grand masters at: waiting.

It was now a wait for the bee and all that blood to say goodbye. Well, to exit her vagina anyway. I think if it had said goodbye on the way out as well we'd have *really* freaked out.

Rosie knew that she had a three-week deadline. She also knew that there was nothing she could do to hurry it along. If it hadn't, er, fallen out by three weeks, there was a procedure she would have to undergo to remove it.

Luckily she had already talked to lots of people about miscarriages and quite a few of them had had the 'procedure'. It's not ideal, they told her, and not very pleasant. Oh, and there's a small risk of it damaging the womb lining and perhaps making it impossible to have a baby in the future. Otherwise fine.

This wait was as bad as all the others.

I quickly decided to block out Eric the Bee and never think of him again.

Instead, I tried to quell all sentiment by actively thinking of him in brutal biological terms: a dead piece of tissue attached to a thick, bloody womb lining that needed to exit my wife via the front bottom.

The bloody reality

For Rosie, the wait was the waiting for her dead embryo to be discharged. That is what she was waiting for and that's what was going to happen.

And the more days that passed, the more uncomfortable and upset she became.

Eventually she WANTED it to come out.

Not just to avoid the potential procedure – which, from what my sister told me, seems to involve a vacuum cleaner sucking the waste products out – but just to reach the end of this nasty chapter.

And to achieve that silly word 'closure' that everyone now uses – as if 'closure' actually exists or means anything and as if everything is okay afterwards. Nothing closes.

But about two and a half weeks later Rosie started the day in a lot of pain. Cramping and a lot of blood. Every hour she had to go to the loo, often having to change her underwear.

Some time around lunchtime I heard a shout. I went upstairs where she wanted me to be with her in the bathroom. She wasn't so much in pain as in shock.

Her eyes were as wide as puddles, she grimaced, writhed and howled.

'Oh God, I think that's it.'

What she would describe as one of the strangest sensations she had ever had had just occurred.

I told her not to look.

It's what they said at the clinic.

They said not to check the remains. They even said that some women reach into the toilet and put the remains in plastic bags and bring the bags into the clinic and demand autopsies. Rather bizarrely, we kind of understood why. They want to know why their baby has died. They want answers. There must be a reason. There just must.

But we remembered what Liz the ultrasound lady said about missing pieces and we did not want to know the reason. Because there would not be one.

Ignoring my growing protestations, Rosie did look.

Fortunately, because our bee was so small there was just blood and uterine discharge all over the toilet and no distinguishable shape. Almost immediately her pain subsided. She flushed the toilet. And there went our bee.

The process of repair

Rather unexpectedly, the whole scarlet extravaganza made Rosie soon feel rather cleansed.

She knew that her womb could now start to repair itself, a sensation which made Rosie feel she could repair herself too.

A woman down the road who Rosie knows came round later that day. She clearly understood the situation and gave Rosie a small, ornamental rose bush. Rosie planted it that afternoon and we never talked about Eric The Bee again.

But we did talk to lots of people about miscarriages. I went out for a drink with a good friend of mine. He has three kids but, it turns out, his wife had a miscarriage between each one. They were even planning a fourth child but she had another miscarriage and couldn't face any more.

I talked to my sister at length, for the first time in probably decades. Finally she told me about her miscarriages, mostly because it was the first time I had ever asked about them.

The first one she had was about 20 years ago, before her daughter was born. The miscarriage was at six months and she had to go to hospital and give birth to a six-month-old baby which she had known for a week was already dead. In fact, so baby-like was it by that stage that it wasn't called a 'miscarriage', but that hideous term, a 'stillborn'.

So now I know about miscarriages, and if you've felt the need to read this chapter, you probably do too.

And since we had ours (or, more correctly, Rosie had hers), whisper it quietly, but I sort of marvel at the strength of the female spirit.

There's a reason men are so shit when they have colds. We really do have a lower pain threshold.

Fuck only knows how we would cope if the one thing we'd been trying to create for years fell out of our bums. We'd have to have a hearse and a shrine, a media blackout, books of condolence, a week's silence and a decade off work.

But ask a woman how she coped with a miscarriage, or several of them, how they coped with the remains of their dead offspring being discharged into the loo and the answer is almost always the same:

'You just do,' they say.

How to survive this stage

* There is no way men can understand what it feels like to be given the news that the thing you have wanted all these years, the thing you finally created whose brand new, little beating heart you actually saw on a TV monitor has now died. There just isn't. But

try to remind her – in the most delicate way possible – that this is nature's ingenious way of filtering out the healthy from the unhealthy. This isn't a baby that was ever meant to be.

* Also remember just how common miscarriages actually are. That means there are a lot of mums and sisters and female friends out there who will have had them and it might be helpful for her (and maybe you) to talk to them.

* Far easier said than done, but try to be there for the actual moment. Rosie – who's pretty tough in the world of females – was really distressed, mentally and physically, and was very grateful to have me there.

* Tell her, urge her, order her (yeah, I know, good luck) not to look at 'it' in the loo or wherever it happens. It is in no way helpful and just creates a visual memory of all the hideousness.

* As soon as humanely possible afterwards, try to get away with her. Go on holiday. Get drunk. Make grand and brilliant plans for the future. Do whatever it takes to get as far away mentally as you can from this strange, unfair, unpredictable world of baby-making. There really is more to life than just trying to create it.

The consultant says...

The vast majority of miscarriages are your body's way of saying that the embryo that got you pregnant just wasn't up to the job.

It's your built-in quality-control mechanism. The first level of quality control is that you won't get pregnant, the second level of quality control is that you miscarry.

It is horribly common but it doesn't necessarily mean that there's an increased chance of it happening again.

Where are you now?

You have had the devastating news that your embryo,
your baby, has died

*

You have either experienced a miscarriage at home
or had an ERPC procedure

*

You have cried a lot

*

You have both coped but probably in different ways

*

You have both discussed a plan for the future,
whether that be trying again or moving on

15

IVF finally works

HER

IVF finally works

Yes, amazingly, with a little bit of luck and a lot of crossed fingers, IVF can and does work.

After the crushing disappointment of a miscarriage it takes a huge almighty effort to face another round of IVF, not to mention a huge almighty scramble to get together the money for a new cycle.

But if you have even the teensiest bit of fight left, your desire to be a mother is still flickering away, and if, of course, the test results are on your side, then you will do your best to find a way.

We did and finally, third time lucky, IVF granted us a successful pregnancy. And that is what this whole book is all about.

As I write this chapter I am approaching 39 weeks of pregnancy.

My baby is wriggling around inside of me and my house is full of babygros, nappies, breast pumps and all the other countless bits of paraphernalia that go with this life-changing event.

As hard as it is to believe, I am at the end of the IVF road and hopefully, you are too.

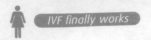

What happened to us

Preparing for a final IVF attempt

So, yeah, despite knocking them at the time, after my failed second attempt at IVF we did what all those 'helpful' people suggested and we got ourselves a dog. A lovely little border terrier called Jeremy (which for some reason seemed like a good idea for a name at the time).

He was such a cute little puppy and was a wonderful happy distraction to take our minds off all the heartache and frustration of the last few years. Poor dog, he must have been completely smothered by all the love we had stored up and he really did (and does) bring so much joy into our hearts.

BUT, he wasn't a baby.

Yes, he was cute and cuddly and funny and sweet but he didn't fill the hole that was left by Eric the Bee. In fact, all that outpouring of love just made me feel that I had so much more to give and that I could be quite good at this mothering thing (now I'd experienced some sleepless nights, frightened cuddles and truly horrific poo incidents).

We had to try again.

We were incredibly lucky in that, because we had moved, we were now in a different health authority and we were able to have our third round of IVF funded by the NHS. I know many people don't have that option and the cost is sometimes just too prohibitive. It is heartbreaking and awful that money plays such a big role in such an emotive situation, but that is one of the things that makes IVF so hard – all those intense emotions and consequences come with a price – a very high price for most people.

With the cost hurdle gratefully sidestepped, it was time to get myself physically and mentally ready.

I resumed acupuncture and hypnotherapy and booked some time off work. I started drinking milk and eating royal jelly with bee pollen (tastes disgusting but it's supposed to help egg quality). I worked on being as relaxed and positive as possible. I wanted to throw everything into this round and put in place all the lessons I'd learnt.

It felt like the final roll of the dice.

Of course, we never said this to each other definitively – that would have been too stressful a situation to address – but I think we both felt it was now or never. That would suggest there was a lot of pressure going into our third cycle but actually we felt pretty calm.

This time we knew what we were doing. We knew what worked for us and what didn't, we'd had the disappointment of a negative result and the joy of a positive, as well as the devastation of a miscarriage. We felt equipped for all eventualities.

When we walked into the consultant's office at yet another clinic for our third (and final) cycle we knew which drug protocol to ask for, which drugs to request and how we wanted the procedures to go.

We knew what to expect from all the key moments, how we'd feel during the two-week wait and how best to relax and keep positive during the whole process.

In other words, we had the benefit of hindsight, something we hope we can pass on with this book so that perhaps your first cycle will be as successful as our third.

Because we believe that with a bit of knowledge and preparation (oh yes, and a lot of luck) there is no reason why IVF can't work first time.

Or, put it this way, IVF is too costly (both financially and emotionally) to leave to trial and error. Hopefully, we've done all the trialling and erroring for you.

I am really pregnant?

After a long time dreaming of this distant concept called pregnancy, when IVF does finally work, it feels pretty unbelievable. Even though I am sitting here, 39 weeks pregnant, I still have the mindset of an 'infertile'.

I'm well aware that it can be hard reading about a pregnancy when you're struggling with infertility and going through IVF.

Some days I would feel intensely angry at anyone who dared walk past me flaunting their smug, round tummy in my face.

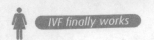

Other days I just felt sad, wondering if I would ever know how it felt to hold my own baby in my arms. And sometimes I would read about a successful IVF pregnancy and feel a surge of hope, proof that it really is possible and does actually work sometimes.

Whatever mood you're in when you read this – if you choose to skip this chapter until you feel like it, that is fine by me – I promise that I get it and I understand.

It certainly wasn't easy getting to this point.

Well, actually, let me re-phrase that, the actual pregnancy has been remarkably easy, physically, and for that I truly feel grateful to my little baby who has been reassuringly normal and average on every scan and check up, making the last nine months substantially easier than they could have been.

But I still managed to make up for it with my own healthy dose of worry and anxiety.

You don't go through years of infertility and three gruelling rounds of IVF and expect pregnancy to be a breeze.

You're hard-wired to expect disappointment and bad news and it takes a while to get your head around the idea that this thing that you've always wanted and dreamed of and fantasised about might actually be happening for you now.

Don't get me wrong. I was happy. Really, really happy. Deep down I was actually incredulous that it had finally worked and this elusive gift of motherhood might soon become a reality. For me. Infertile, low-AMH me. Over 35 years old, never-been-pregnant me.

My very own child.

I could at last make those forbidden daydreams a reality. Playing with my little splashing baby in the bath, getting the giggles on the swings, holding hands in the park. Could all this really come true? For me? After all this time? It was so incredible that I just couldn't quite believe it. For ages.

The first few months

The first three months dragged slowly.

I had all the symptoms, some quite potent morning sickness (well, mine was more evening sickness), sore boobs, headaches and shoulder pains.

I had a scan at the clinic at seven weeks which confirmed a heartbeat flickering away and then had another scan at nine weeks where we saw the heartbeat again and more of a bean-shaped blob – basically more like what we should have seen at our devastating ten-week scan the second time around.

The words that changed everything

It was this nine-week scan that made all the difference for us.

Partly because we had now got further along than ever before and we were past the point where it had all gone wrong last time but mostly because the lady scanning me said something I will remember forever.

Richard started asking her about odds and percentages of things going wrong after this point (that's how we had come to talk after years of IVF procedures) and she just said 'oh, don't worry, that's a nice strong heartbeat, you'll be fine with this one now.'

She was a little bit older than most of the IVF nurses we'd encountered, a bit less clinical than we were used to and perhaps a bit less worried about following the careful language code that seems drilled into all IVF professionals, to avoid giving false hope.

But she didn't realise what a huge impact her words had on us.

Throughout all three cycles no one had ever said anything like that.

It had all been a case of 'well, of course you're making good progress but anything can happen, there are no guarantees, sometimes we don't know why things stop developing, chromosomes, genetics, blah blah blah'.

You were constantly aware that you were dealing with a scientific process that was far removed from the world of human reassurance and empathy.

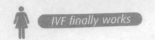

Of course, people had been kind and gentle but they had always been careful to only deal with the pure hard facts and figures. No one had ever really stuck their neck out and said what they REALLY thought was going on.

And that was why it was just so lovely to hear from an experienced sonographer that she thought we had a keeper. No caveats, no backtracking, just a really nice, genuine, reassuring few words that we kept with us the whole pregnancy.

We are so grateful to that woman.

There should be more of that in the world of IVF. I completely understand the reluctance to dish out false hope but where you do see some positive signs, is there really that much harm in vocalising them to your couples? If not, why not?

We're not so stupid as to blame that woman if it had gone wrong – we wouldn't sue her for what she said or raise a complaint.

We'd just know that nothing can be certain and things do go wrong, as we'd been told countless times. But at least for that short time we'd have had a little bit more hope and positivity surrounding us. Surely that's no bad thing?

The 12-week scan

Of course, although that nine-week scan felt like a milestone there were still plenty more hoops to go through.

We had our NHS 12-week scan and I remember being petrified to look at the screen during that one in case there was no heartbeat.

But yet again, baby came up trumps and there it was, that beautiful, tiny, pulsating light flickering away. This time we could hear it and that was a truly wonderful sound.

I was still cautious, for reasons I'll fully explain below, but I did finally feel that I was nearly there and almost able to start believing in my little growing bean.

The next hoop to get through was the test for Down's Syndrome.

After the 12-week scan, the NHS send you your chances of the baby having Down's (by now we were more than used to odds and chances and percentages of survival).

Our odds came back at 1/460 – low enough for the NHS not to worry about it but high enough for me to.

We didn't fancy the invasive tests but found there is a new one on the market called the Harmony Test. It is just a blood test, but it is a bit more accurate than the current NHS test and can actually test for chromosome markers in the baby, carried in the mother's blood.

But, of course, we had to pay for this test and again I was so grateful that we could afford to do so. It cost us about £500 at a private London clinic, where they threw in a scan at the same time to check all the physical developmental factors. Expensive, but incredibly reassuring when our Down's odds eventually came back at 1:10,000.

This scan at about 15 weeks was amazing and was the first time we could really see our baby in detail. The sonographer showed us all the limbs and organs and it actually all started to make sense. She even took a guess at the sex but couldn't be certain so we had to hang on until the 20-week scan for that.

Trying to come to terms with it

All this time I kept a mental distance from the pregnancy.

I knew it was all going okay, I felt sick for at least 16 weeks but I sort of processed it more like, 'Gosh, I'm feeling unwell at the moment', rather than progressing my pregnancy. I just couldn't properly engage with it. I desperately wanted to but there must have been a great big subconscious block in the way.

Every scan was a hurdle that I could jump over but after each one when the initial elation subsided I went back to my same slightly numb state and looked towards the next hurdle to start the worrying again.

It became quite frustrating, not just for me but also for Richard.

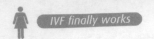

He couldn't understand that I had wanted to be pregnant for so, so long and now it was here I didn't seem that excited or pleased or even that happy to talk about it.

Feeling the heartbeat

Then we had the NHS 20-week scan and found out that we were having a little girl.

Soon after that I began to feel the first flutterings of movement and started to properly show the beginnings of a little round bump.

Suddenly it all clicked into place.

That black cloud that I had been so used to living under for so long, suddenly, as though because of a refreshing gust of wind, just blew away and was replaced by a wonderful lightness that has stayed with me the whole pregnancy. The sense of relief was overwhelming.

I didn't have to hold my breath until the next scan for proof that my baby's heart was still beating – I could just put my hand on my tummy and feel a little flutter of movement and get that instant reassurance. And that made all the difference to me.

I could also start visualising the little girl she would become.

A girl. My little girl. My daughter.

I had been happy for it to be a boy or a girl, of course, but I was so delighted to be having a little girl and actually sort of had an inkling that that was what it would be. It's funny that they say you just know.

I dared myself to imagine what she might look like, think about those baby girl names we'd had rattling around all those years and even started talking to her, rubbing my belly as I spoke.

We had a holiday in Spain (our first holiday abroad for three years) and we would spend the days sunbathing and marvelling at the wriggles and bumps in my tummy. Finally we both really started connecting with the baby and talking about it as though it really was going to happen.

I am extremely lucky to have a very active little baby, she moves a lot and I'm so very grateful for that.

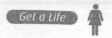

A normal, pregnant woman

After the 20-week scan I felt like I could and indeed should start telling people. Besides, I couldn't really hide my podgy tummy for much longer.

It was strange telling people at first.

I really didn't want anyone to know – again, it was a self-protection mechanism from the miscarriage when I'd had to tell everyone who knew about the IVF that it had all gone wrong.

So I started telling people the long sorry saga of IVF as if to say, 'yes, I am pregnant but don't go thinking this has been easy for me – it's been a struggle and you need to know that'.

Of course, people didn't need to know that and clearly felt uncomfortable, as if I was asking them to temper their congratulations.

Eventually, however, I learnt to just accept a 'great, congrats' for what it was and not have to go into all the gory detail of how it came to pass.

And after a while, I began to feel like a normal pregnant person who perhaps hadn't been through all of the shit to get there. I didn't forget, of course, but I'd bid that dark cloud adieu and was just so happy to be pregnant at last.

I was no longer a strange social outcast – the one who doesn't have kids yet, the one who couldn't be invited to a christening, the one who talks about her dog like it's her baby. Weirdo. I was just a pregnant woman.

Even the doctors didn't seem that interested in it being an IVF pregnancy, I was treated as normal, low-risk, having-a-very-average bog-standard pregnancy. Ah, the joys of being considered average.

The legacy of IVF

Of course, I still have my moments.

I still feel like a fraud in Baby Gap, even now I keep thinking I'll be 'found out'.

I still wake up in the morning and have a shudder of panic before I feel a friendly little kick that allows me to continue with my day. And I don't take any of it for granted, not for one moment.

But despite the worries and self-doubt, I can honestly say I have really

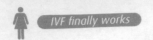

enjoyed being pregnant. I have loved my changing body, even though I do look like Mr Greedy, according to Richard.

I have felt glorious despite the swollen ankles, heartburn and bouts of blue hands (my own special pregnancy symptom).

I have loved reading, researching, preparing and nesting.

What I didn't realise was that everyone is so nice to you when you're pregnant, it's as though you exude this special glow that makes people want to be kind and generous. No, not everyone is happy to give up their seat on the Tube for you, but people send you special smiles and ask you how it's going and when you're due.

Of course, everyone has an opinion about how you should be feeling, how awful birth will be and a million theories on the best way to get babies to sleep through the night, but I have let it all wash over me and found my own way.

And that's part of the legacy of IVF.

Something so precious and longed-for has finally been gifted to me and I'm not going to let anyone ruin it.

Richard and I will make lots of mistakes and no doubt do many things people find weird or wrong, but we will do it together and we will find our own way.

We're just so grateful we've been given the opportunity to do this and that finally, after all our fertility ups and downs, it actually bloody worked.

And that is the most miraculous, amazing, surprising and wonderful thing about IVF.

Sometimes, it actually works.

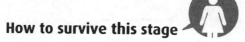

How to survive this stage

* Take each day at a time – try not to look too far ahead – either positively or negatively.

* See each scan/test/check up as a hurdle and celebrate getting over each one.

* If you're finding it hard to bond with your growing baby perhaps write a diary to record your feelings and 'talk' to your bump.

* Keep your pregnancy tests and scan pictures somewhere you can see them daily – there will be many times you won't believe it's all happening so it will help to provide visual reassurance.

* Speak to other people who've been through IVF successfully – it will help you believe that you too can be part of this camp.

* Ignore the horror stories/vitriolic advice. Know that you will do things your way.

* When you're ready, make sure you embrace your pregnancy. I know that I may only do this once so I wanted to make sure I did everything I wanted to do. This ranged from having an expensive pregnancy massage to having professional maternity bump photos taken to having the best milkshake in London (my particular third-trimester craving).

* Take time to enjoy being with your partner (and dog!) and really enjoy the last few months of being a couple before your worlds get turned upside down.

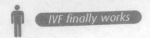
HIM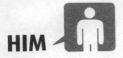

IVF finally works

Much like I hoped you wouldn't need to read the last chapter, I hope you find yourself needing to read this one.

Not because it's full of startling insight or wonderful prose, but just because it proves that all the horror and hideousness I've cacked on about in the last 14 chapters is worth it.

Despite all the pressure and arguments and madness and even though the odds are against you right from the beginning, I can assure you IVF does work.

And when it works it tends to result in the creation of a miniature human.

I know this because there's one inside my wife as I write this and this chapter is everything you need to know about what is a very odd few months.

What happened to us

Hopefully you'll be reading this at the culmination of your first (and only) attempt at IVF.

But even if it's your second or third or however many, it doesn't matter, the process is the same:

- She'll wee on her stick.

- She'll have her first scan about three weeks later.

- You'll see a little pulsating bean on a screen.

- She might have a scan at about 9–10 weeks to check everything is okay but, more commonly you'll wait until 12–13 weeks and there, on the screen is a miniature, see-through human.

- Your life will never be the same ever again.

Discovering there's an actual baby this time

Because it was the third (and probably final) time we would do IVF, and because on our second round of IVF our embryo had died at around the seven–eight week mark, the nine-week scan obviously had slightly bigger ramifications for us.

Just to recap our little fertility tale:

- **Start trying to conceive**: Summer 2007
- **Tried really hard to conceive:** July 2008
- **Starting arguing a lot**: June 2009
- **Carried on arguing**: July 2009–February 2010
- **Started investigative tests**: May 2010
- **1st IVF attempt** October 2011: Two embryos put back but pregnancy test negative
- **2nd IVF attempt**: March 2012: Two embryos put back and a positive pregnancy test but embryo dies at about eight weeks
- **3rd IVF attempt**: February 2013: One embryo put back, positive pregnancy test, and a miniature human is created, with a due date of October 2013

Moving a bit further forward each time

What kept Rosie going through those five years – apart from the, by now, rabid desire to have a baby and be like ALL THOSE OTHER WOMEN – was the fact that at each stage of IVF we went a little bit further.

- **1st IVF attempt:** A complete no-show.
- **2nd IVF attempt:** Pregnant for the first time ever in her life.
- **3rd IVF attempt:** Pregnant again and hoping to baby Jesus that it wouldn't curl up and die this time.

After the great eye-opener that was the bloody world of miscarriage at the end of our second attempt, the third time we did IVF the early scans were a very different affair.

Seven-week scan: the throbbing bean

After the positive pregnancy stick we went back to the clinic – another, different clinic as we'd moved house in the meantime – and saw the little pulsating bean.

Small, indistinct and throbbing. Relief and quiet, tempered joy, but no silly names this time.

Nothing that might create too memorable an attachment. This time the photo of that monochrome bean stayed in its cardboard folder in a drawer with all the forms and didn't make it on to the fridge.

Nine-week scan: the moment of truth

This time there are no silly jokes about the embryo not being there, just a terrified silence as we drive back to the clinic. After the imagined life I would share with Eric the Bee, I had realised how much I actually cared about this process.

Rosie, meanwhile, was, quite simply, absolutely shitting her pants.

We didn't plan or legislate for a second time, let alone a third and since the miscarriage, the tense and tone of our conversation had subtly changed.

I noticed now that Rosie's clause had changed from 'when we have a baby we will...' to 'if we don't have a baby we could...'

This was a massive mental realignment.

It's a survival mechanism, of course, a means of keeping slightly sane. But it meant that she had finally confronted the possibility that she might never actually have children.

There would be no fourth attempt.

We continued to sit in silence in the waiting area at the clinic, trying hard to avoid the stares of the dozens of babies all over the walls. I mean, photos of babies, not actual babies – as that would just be weird. And probably illegal.

It's one of the strange things that united all three clinics where we did IVF: in the waiting area, yes, there'll be comfy seats and varying qualities of coffee, but there are also always photos of babies everywhere.

It's partly to reinforce the clinic's track record, of course, a little two-dimensional boast of just how good they are at playing God ('oh yeah, this is what we can do with your spunk that you clearly weren't able to manage') and partly, I suppose, to make you feel like it will work and all be okay in the end.

But I can tell you, when you're on your way out of the clinic after being told your embryo is dead you do have an unbelievable urge to give each of those dozens of little pink faces a massive punch.

Someone in a mauve clinician's outfit called our names.

The moment we realised we'd finally made it

We went into a room that had become a bit too familiar and we were greeted by another nice ultrasound lady.

I was relieved to see that she was slightly older than most. Late fifties, I'm guessing. I like late fifties or early sixties in IVF, It suggests loads of experience and when they say something good or bad it means they've seen hundreds of similar situations and know what they're talking about.

Rosie was barely able to take off her jeans for shaking. She gripped my hand like she was strangling a fish and lay down.

There was that long pause.

The nice ultrasound lady had a feel around Rosie's insides with her magic, moisturised wand.

Another pause.

Blackness on the TV screen and the thump of Rosie's heart.

'There it is,' said the nice ultrasound lady and Rosie's hand-strangle eased.

Of course, Rosie wanted complete reassurance and wanted to know if it looked healthy (= is this one going to die and ruin the rest of my life?).

'Well, that's one hell of a heartbeat pumping away there and I don't think you'll have any problems with this one.'

It was a sentence we were so grateful to hear and a sentence that would help us sleep over the next few weeks.

Rosie made a noise of audible relief.

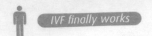

Her bundle of throbbing cells was now nine weeks old. She knew that with each day the odds would improve massively.

She also knew that the 12-week scan would be back in a normal hospital, a normal NHS hospital where normal women who think they're pregnant after having normal sex go for scans.

12-week scan: meeting your alien offspring

And so, eight weeks after that fraught and fretful early morning wee and about five years since this strange and hideous experience began, we went to our local NHS hospital and finally Rosie had become a normal pregnant woman, a patient number on an NHS maternity database.

Unfortunately, Ridley Scott rather ruined the great magic and mystery of pregnancy for me.

I was too young when I first saw the famous John Hurt scene in *Alien*, I think about eight years old; old enough to love the gore and the space scenes but young enough to never quite be comfortable with the idea of things living inside humans. And, be warned, the 12-week scan does nothing to ease this.

This time on the TV screen you see an alien, not a child. A writhing, kicking, translucent alien living inside the abdomen of the woman you love. You can see through its skin and bones. The chainlink Meccano of its spine. You can see right into its brain. You can actually see its thoughts.

We were overjoyed and relieved and all those things, make no mistake, but there really is nothing cute about this moment.

This time a quiet and efficient ultrasound nurse was pressing the handset on that gel stuff on Rosie's stomach (no need for the wand up the vag this time). She kept freezing the image and measuring things and making notes. Very perfunctory, almost bored.

It was oddly reassuring that everything was average and fine and boring.

But suddenly I managed to surmount my alien-based mental blockage of a see-through parasite living in my wife's guts, as I noticed the see-through thing had fingers.

Actual fingers.

And toes.

Tiny toes on the end of actual legs.

And you could see its forehead and nose and the profile of its eyes and it moved around and appeared to be facing us.

It was looking at me. And my only thought was 'Jesus Christ, now I REALLY need to get a job'.

The scary photo

We got some photos of the see-through thing – £3 each, well, it is the NHS – and on the way back to the car I had a look at them and, saying nothing, handed them to Rosie. She had a look at them and said nothing.

'Did you notice it?' I said, eventually.

'What?' she said.

'You know... the, er...'

'The nose?'

'Yes, the nose.'

'Course I did. Do you think it's a mistake?'

Now, I have a slightly dominant nose, not huge, just slightly prominent. A little pointy, perhaps. Sometimes it's bigger than others. Sometimes I don't notice it at all and other times I see a reflection or a photo and it looks ridiculous. But, after four decades on the planet, I'm used to it. It's an heirloom, of course, kindly passed down by my father and all his fathers. Noses run in my family, as it were.

But this thing on these photos is HUGE.

Not so much a nose, more a beak.

We'd heard about those occasional mix-ups in embryology labs – they're always well publicised – when white parents find themselves giving birth to black children and black parents giving birth to white children and so on – but we'd never heard of them mixing the eggs and sperms up with that of a toucan.

The thing had a beak.

On every photo.

An elongated triangle designed for pecking coming out of its face.

So the first one was a bee, and this one was a bird?

Why didn't the ultrasound woman mention it?

Was she just being polite?

Did she not want to draw attention to my unfortunate nasal genes?

The 4D scam

The next scan was at 20 weeks, which checked for a load of things we were shitting ourselves about, even though the odds of our baby having them were almost the same as being born with a beak.

And then, well, just because, Rosie decided to pay for a private scan at about the 28-week stage.

She'd heard about a thing called '4D' scans where they can print off an accurate image of the baby rather than just a grainy black and white see-through thing. However, we both knew tacitly that she was doing it to check the progress of the beak.

Just a tip, if your good lady tells you about 4D scans and how you should definitely have one because it'll be a really nice thing to have and it's an important stage, etc., etc., stand up (if you're not standing up already), tell her she's wrong and that everything she's saying is horse shit. Then sit down again.

For the record, we have a 4D image, incredibly reasonably priced, as you'd imagine, and it looks like a semi-melted waxwork of John Merrick covered in trifle.

And while we're on it, why '4D'? Surely '2D'? It's a piece of paper with the smudge of a flattened human on it. That's not even three dimensions. And still women fall for this crap.

Luckily, at the same scan, we got the usual, grainy, two-dimensional black and white ones.

We checked them, de rigueur, on the way back to the car.

Oh, thank God.

The beak was just a printing error. Or it had fallen off. Who cares? In its place was a tiny, snub baby nose of the type usually seen on 28-week old babies in wombs.

Doing it yourself: turning into a cliché

There's not much else you need to know.

It's all covered in about 5000 books on pregnancy, some of which will appear in your home around this time, that you will never read and never need to read.

What's odd is how boring and normal it all makes you feel and how oddly reassuring that sensation is.

You will occasionally think you are the first people on Earth to have created a baby but then you realise you're probably the 7,246,611,104th and people have been doing it for about 150,000 years.

Like lots of women, Rosie had morning sickness which was never before lunch time and didn't result in nausea but made her feel pretty dreadful every day. But it was only for the first few months and she never moaned about it because, given what we'd been through, it just wasn't something that needed to be moaned about.

Meanwhile, I turned into a ludicrous home improvement cliché.

This initially meant venturing into The Room.

The Room was one of the strangest things in our lives.

We'd moved from a flat to a house and there was a spare room. When we moved in it was generally referred to as The Baby's Room, but as we started to come to terms with the possibility that there may be no baby it just became The Room.

As we struggled through the various pits of IVF hell, The Room came to symbolise everything that was going wrong.

This space, this gap, this unused emptiness in our lives; hopelessly unfilled and unused. We started to just dump things in there to make it less empty. After two years you could barely open the door, which wasn't such a problem as neither of us could really bear to go in there.

But now it was time to tackle The Room.

A shame really to get rid of the dark pond-green paint the previous owners had smeared all over the walls, and a shame to have to tell each of my 106 carrier bags of cassettes and CDs and Important Bits Of Paper that they would have to find a new home, but such was our new now.

And I turned into something terrible from an advert.

Having never owned a paintbrush or a screwdriver I now began sanding things and varnishing things and stripping and painting and recoating. I'd never even done any DIY in my life and now I'd turned into this.

Rosie's friends would come round and she'd proudly show off this interior transformation. 'Oh, he's nesting' I could hear them say.

'I'm not "nesting" it's called "decorating"' I would scream, inches from their faces, as I tore their heads from their necks in the paint fumes of my mind, my fury rising as I confronted the horrible reality that I had become one of those expectant, worried, first-time dads I'd detested all these years.

After five years of people messing with our bits and our minds, and all that torment and intrusion and despair and humiliation and w-a-i-t-i-n-g, endless waiting, we were finally normal.

Like other people.

Before turning the lights out we now just marvel at this thing growing inside Rosie. At the 20-week scan we knew it was a girl. And each night, at almost exactly the same time, she kicks and prods and visibly stretches the skin of Rosie's stomach. They actually kick. I mean, we all hear this stuff, but, fuck, they really do. And hard. A seven-month-old girl with a wonderful career ahead of her in kick-boxing or swimming or Irish dancing.

And everything else they tell you that you will go through – all that fear and wonder – is all true too.

Finally we've made it and we're amazed and scared and boring and normal.

Of course we are.

We always were.

That's why they call IVF 'assisted conception', because that's really all it is. A bit of help to get to a place that other people take for granted.

But I'll shut up now because if you've got this far in the book you'll know all this, or will do soon, and be as soppy and boring as me.

You've made it. Congratulations. You're going to be a parent.

Now begins the *really* difficult bit....

How to survive this stage

* She will still be worried about how the baby is doing – and there are delightful tests (and more odds), like the one for Down's syndrome, but you both know that after that 12-week scan the odds are finally on your side.

* Be aware that the 12-week scan is scary and unsettling. Or perhaps it was just me...?

* Don't waste your money on the '4D' scans. Just imagine a fetus covered in butter and mud and it's the same thing.

* Be wary of the photos of the scans, particularly if they appear to show odd protuberances, such as beaks.

* And, to be honest, the surviving bit is finally over. Just enjoy the fact you've finally got here and try to get as much sleep now as you can possibly fit in....

The consultant says...

The thing to remember is that every single pregnancy is different – every woman will respond differently.

Some women will have absolutely no symptoms, other women will have the worst morning sickness ever.

The main thing is not to get stressed out if you don't have the symptoms that so many women talk about.

Where are you now?

You are feeling a bit better

*

She starts seeing your friends with babies again

*

You find yourself forgetting what an ordeal IVF was

*

You are grateful for every kick, hiccup and bout of nausea

*

She can't believe she's legitimately shopping for baby clothes

*

You finally feel like a normal couple about to have a baby

*

You are shit-scared

16

What we learnt from doing IVF

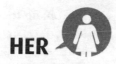

HER

What we learnt from doing IVF

Doing IVF three times was tough, exhausting and undoubtedly the worst few years of my life so far (which, of course, may say more about how lucky I've been rather than how bad IVF was).

But IVF has taught me some valuable life lessons.

Going to the darkest places in my mind and having those feelings of despair certainly puts things in perspective and encourages you to see things a bit differently.

Generally, it has made me more appreciative, more empathetic and less controlling.

And it has taught me to live more for the moment and worry less about the past or the future. Who'd have thought IVF could be so Zen?

I never want to go back to that time but I can now see what it taught me and be grateful for that instead of resenting it.

Ten lessons learnt from doing IVF

1. Don't try to plan your life

I think every woman loves to plan, and what better a thing to plan than your life and how you see it mapping out in front of you?

I'd always dreamt of marriage and family and I used to think, okay, worst-case scenario: as long as I've met my man by the time I'm 30, I will be married by the time I'm 32 then have my first baby at 34 and my second at 36.

Perfect.

I'll still be a relatively yummy mummy and have ticked all the boxes before my fertility falls off a cliff. But it didn't work out like that.

I met Richard when I was 27 but it took us five years to work up to marriage. I guess I still met my 'age-32' deadline, but that's when the plan ceased to work.

Having finally achieved a pregnancy and miscarriage at the age of 36, I am now finally having my first baby at the age of 37 – a few years off my target and I may well have scuppered any chance of having another baby.

During this process I have had to have a complete rethink about my goals.

What would it mean to me if I could only have one child or possibly none?

I have had to confront that scenario as I've seen my self-imposed deadlines come and go. Now, when I hear my friends planning their lives I shudder. 'Things may not work out like that!' I want to shout.

When it comes to your fertility you can't take anything for granted.

Yes, you may fall pregnant on your first attempt but it also may not be like they warned about at school; it could take several months, or even years and by then your small target window will have closed and you'll kick yourself for counting on it.

Basically, anything can happen.

You or your partner might have a serious fertility issue, or you might get knocked down by a bus. Or a lorry. Who knows? Nothing is certain, especially when it comes to fertility.

So stop planning and start being more instinctive. My advice for anyone who knows they want to be a mother someday is to go for it as soon as you practically can (jobs, money and partner permitting).

Don't wait. There will never be a right time. Get on with it.

2. Patience

The biggest lesson to learn when fertility doesn't go your way is how to take a deep breath and wait. And wait. And wait some more.

IVF is all about patience.

You have to wait to get started, perhaps wait to get on the NHS list, wait while you take the drugs and slowly build up your follicles, wait while you see if the process has worked and then a final wait even if it has worked to see if it's viable.

That's not to mention the following nine months during which you actually wait to give birth.

And if it all goes wrong (and you decide to have another go), well you have to pick yourself up and start all over again, like a high-stakes game of Snakes and Ladders.

All the time you can't do anything to speed it up, you must just sit tight and wait... and wait.

I've always been quite impatient, wanting to do things NOW, but since doing IVF, I am extremely patient because I've had to learn to be.

3. Gratitude

One of the ways I stopped spiralling into depression during the dark times after the failed cycle and the miscarriage was to write a gratitude diary.

Yes, I know it's a bit naff and the sort of suggestion you get in self-help books, but it actually worked for me.

The idea is to write down five things every day that you are grateful for.

It could be as simple as 'husband cooked my favourite spaghetti Bolognese again' or 'had a lovely chat with my friend' or even 'got the last seat on the train this morning'.

Whatever your day held, pick out five things that were good.

Then, miraculously, what happens is you start looking out for good, happy things as you go about your day so you can write them in your book.

This means you are now primed to notice good things and be grateful for them immediately. Which makes for a happier day-to-day experience. Simple!

4. All things will pass

You can't see this when you're in the throes of a miscarriage but the dark days will lift, one way or another.

That pain you're experiencing at the moment can't go on forever. I know it feels like it will, but it won't. You WILL get back to your normal self and have happier days in the future.

If you can hold this nugget close to your heart it may just help you get through the heartache.

You don't need to 'snap out of it' or dampen your grief or sadness now, but if you can foresee a time when you will be out of this tunnel, that might help.

I used to think that when I'm 45 all this will be over. I'll either have children or I won't and if I don't I will at least be over it.

I will be through the minefield of my fertile years and my friends' kids will all be older and at school and it won't be the centre of everyone's lives as much as it is now and I will have made my peace with it.

5. Stop comparing yourself to your friends

A lot of these fertile years are about fitting in.

I didn't want to be pregnant at age 25 and I'm guessing I won't really want to be at age 45, but at age 35 it is what all my friends were doing.

I remember there being a time when I was doing IVF when I could count at least 15 people I knew who were pregnant. That's a lot of Facebook to avoid.

When all you see are scan pictures and birth announcements and happy, cosy families you can begin to feel just a little bit left out. For women it starts when you hit 30 and goes on for a good ten years, with the last five being increasingly hysterical as people cram in their second and third babies while you're still struggling to get the first one to appear.

It is a terrible thing to admit that there is an element of wanting to fit in and have kids 'because everyone else is doing it', but it would be naïve to think that is not at least part of the story.

Thirty-somethings don't go to nightclubs or festivals, they have playdates and barbecues with the kids. If you don't have a squealing, drooling three-foot-high appendage you're not really welcome.

It's not because people don't try to make an effort with you, but because it's awkward for everyone.

You can lose a lot of friends during this time so it's useful if you can just park them for a bit. It's hard on you both to make things work, so maybe just know that you'll pick up with them again when this phase is over.

6. Adapt (no, not adopt, adApt)

Okay, so you're infertile. You thought things were going to go one way but they've gone another. You had that lovely image of two kids and picnics on the beach firmly embedded in your head and now the crazy bitch of infertility has slashed it into bits.

All that remains is you and your partner with a handful of dreams to rethink. And so you must.

Perhaps life won't turn out the way you thought, but perhaps it might be better?

I found that only when I could face the worst and imagine what our lives would be without children, could I actually find a bit of joy day to day. It took me a while to confront the idea of childlessness but once I had, it really helped.

I re-shaped the dream with our dog, with travel and nice holidays and exciting careers and perhaps having children in my life in some other way.

I had a vague notion of volunteer teaching or something similar.

For a not-very-adaptable person this was a very liberating way of getting some positivity back into my life. Oh, and yes, of course some people adapt their dreams of having biological children by considering adoption and enriching many lives as a result.

7. Learn to let go

Everyone will tell you the IVF myths: 'so-and-so did five IVF attempts then finally gave up and they got pregnant naturally, age 42!'

Yes, yes, yes, we've all heard those before and they are obscenely unhelpful when you've just had another unsuccessful IVF cycle.

But again, like all myths and clichés there probably is an element of truth in there.

The more you tense up and will yourself through gritted teeth to grow those follicles and implant that embryo, the less likely it seems to be to work. God knows why. One day they will figure out the mind/body connection but until then all we know is to be relaxed is the best possible state you can be in.

Trust that your body will work with the drugs and that, given a little bit of medical help, it knows what to do.

Once you walk through the clinic door you have to leave it to the experts.

They choose your drugs protocol, they scan you, make adjustments and carry out the procedures. You can know everything there is to know to the finite chromosome, but ultimately the outcome is in their hands.

Of course, ask questions and understand what is happening to you and be informed but don't try to control IVF. Don't fight it. Just let your body go with it and stay positive during the process.

Take it from me, this is hard for one with tendencies towards control-freakery.

8. Never take baby for granted

If you are successful and go on to have a 'live birth' (still a horrible phrase) then you will be forever grateful to IVF and the wonders of modern science.

I've seen many harassed mothers over the years and I wouldn't dare to judge any of them, it is a ferociously hard and unforgiving role.

But there is a common thread with all the women I've known who've struggled with infertility.

They never forget the journey they've been through and even when their child is screaming a tantrum in the supermarket and turning purple, they tend to remember, 'I wanted this so much, I went through so much, I must embrace these moments along with the treasured cuddles and love'.

I don't know if they feel this consciously but it seems that mothers who've battled fertility hard for this prize never forget the struggle and don't take their child for granted.

9. Empathy

As a good fellow infertile friend once said, 'We are but foot soldiers in the war on infertility'

And often it really does feel like a war; only those who've been through it can know the true extent of the battle scars.

I feel deep empathy for women and men struggling with infertility and even more for those who've been down the IVF route. No one knows what it's like until you've done it. And if you've had it fail, you know the dark places people have had to go to, particularly to pick themselves up and try again.

Partly the reason for writing this book is to reach out to others going through the same thing and say 'I know how you feel. And it's bloody awful'.

There are no guarantees and nothing I can really say to make it better, but only that I know how you feel and I really truly empathise.

It helps to talk about what a strange mix of emotions it all is – anger, resentment, jealousy, exhaustion, fear, etc., etc. They're all valid and some so dark you can only discuss them with people who have been through it all themselves and know how hard you're struggling behind the exhausted façade of day-to-day life.

10. Just be nice to each other

If you can get through IVF together then you have a pretty special relationship.

Research has suggested that IVF is as stressful as divorce or having cancer in the family, so you are going to go through some tough times together. Never mind the indignity of the scans or the pain of injections and weird hormones, there are just some horrible emotional scenes that are headed your way.

You may not always have the same view about it all, particularly how much of your life (and money) you are going to devote to IVF. And if you go through a failed cycle or a miscarriage there will be great sadness and grief to get through together – which may happen at a different pace.

There may also be blame or resentment or guilt – depending on who bears the brunt of the fertility issues. Most couples never need to address anywhere near these levels of difficult emotions so don't despair if you find it tricky.

But for all that, there will be great tenderness and love as you support each other through it all and share the excitement and ups and downs on this emotional journey.

Be kind to each other. If IVF doesn't tear you apart it will most certainly bring you together and you will feel stronger as a result.

If you can get through this together, you will certainly be able to get through most other life hurdles too. I've heard the first few months with a newborn can be tough on your relationship.

After IVF, it will be a breeze.

HIM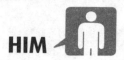

What we learnt from doing IVF

If you flip over to 'Her' version of this chapter you'll find ten heartfelt and moving life lessons which Rosie learnt from the whole IVF journey ('Oh God, he just called it a "journey". What a wanker.')

Perhaps because I'm not fitted with female parts or because I'm just a nasty bag of old bollocks, I don't feel like this.

What did I learn from IVF?

Well, it's expensive, incredibly draining, stressful, unpredictable, hard on relationships, humiliating and strange.

But you'll know all that from the last 15 chapters.

Instead, having done IVF three times I now realise just how different it is to natural conception and why people who haven't done IVF just don't understand what we (and you) have been through.

To highlight just how different it is, overleaf is a helpful table comparing the two at each key stage:

IVF v natural conception

STAGE	IVF	Natural conception
DECIDE TO HAVE CHILDREN	Have sex but nothing happens	Get drunk and bang her on the sofa
	Chart ovulation dates and start having sex at precise times	Have sex in the mornings before work
	Improve diet, do more exercise, stop drinking alcohol and have sex at even more precise times	Take her roughly from behind on back seat of car
	Start avoiding sex as you realise you hate having sex with each other	Go to music festival, get wankered and go like the clappers in a hedge
	Make appointment with GP and do tests for semen quality	Get fellated on sofa
	Do lots of other tests and begin IVF treatment, injecting her legs each evening with follicle-stimulating hormones	Have so much sex that you actually bruise your member
CONCEIVE CHILD	Wank in a booth and hand semen sample to nurse	Have even more sex, including Waitrose car park and in the toilets at Cafe Pasta
	Wait nervously at home for fertilisation results	Watch DVD box set with intermittent sex
	Receive regular updates on embryo development and go back to clinic for embryo transfer	Go on holiday, drink revolting local liquor and perform violent cunnilingus while bent double on elderly German couple's rented Prius
	Wait nervously for two weeks, trying to remain busy and upbeat	Return from holiday and wait while she clears up her vaginal thrush
PREGNANCY TEST	She wees on a stick having not slept for two nights and checks the pregnancy testing kit 53 times, leaps triumphantly around bedroom and tells everyone she's ever met that she's finally pregnant	Go to work, go to pub, see friends, have a nice walk

PREGNANCY SCANS	Three weeks later, go to clinic for first scan and, while she trembles nervously, see 9 mm embryo on screen and stare amazed at heartbeat	She tells you she can't remember the last time she had her period. You're part pleased, part terrified, then she goes off to work
	Three weeks after last scan go back to clinic and repeat process to make sure embryo is still alive and developing	Go and see new film at independent cinema, eat out at new Thai restaurant, go to something pretentiously highbrow at local arts centre
	Two–three weeks later go for first scan at NHS hospital and marvel at every detail	Get dragged along to see first scan at NHS hospital
	About four weeks after that, pay for a 16-week panic scan just to make sure everything is still okay then celebrate tentatively, aware that this is very far from the end of the journey	She starts getting annoyed that she can't get drunk
	Four weeks later, go to NHS hospital for routine 20-week scan to discover gender of baby. Cry with joy if it's a boy. If it's a girl, also cry with joy.	Have discussion about merits of boy v girl. Get bit annoyed that it's not a boy. Then console yourself that little boys just break things and piss everywhere.
AT 9 MONTHS	Prepare for big day and realise life will never be the same again. Sort out spare room.	Prepare for big day and realise life will never be the same again. Sort out spare room.

The consultant says...

I think the ultimate lesson of IVF is that you can never be in complete control.

No one has a right to a successful fertility outcome. All you can do is try to control the things you can in terms of maximising success.

All fertility clinics can do is try to optimise the building blocks that you give us, but we can't control everything.

Where are you now?

You have done it

*

You have actually made a baby

*

You have got through one of the hardest periods of
your lives together

*

You have now just like any other average couple with a baby

*

IVF will soon seem like a strange, needle-filled, distant memory

*

Congratulations

*

Now buy all that baby stuff and get all the sleep
you possibly can

Questions you need to ask at the consultation

These questions are repeated from pages 69–71 for you to tear out and take with you on your consultation.

1. What drugs will I be on?

(Required for down-regulation, stimulation and triggering the release of the eggs – there is a more detailed explanation of all these in the next chapter.)

- What dose will I be on and why?

- How do I administer the drugs – are they all by injection or do I sniff the down-regulation drug?

- When will I be shown how to mix up and inject the drugs?

- Can I source the drugs myself or must I buy them from your pharmacy?

2. What is the timeline?

- How soon can I start?

- On what day of my cycle do I start the down-regulation drugs and how long am I on them for?

- When is my baseline scan to assess that all is shut down and quiet? When will I start taking the stimulating drugs and how long (on average) after stimulating is the egg collection?

3. How often will I have monitoring scans/blood tests?

(Not all clinics do blood tests.)

- How flexible are the scanning appointments (i.e., do you have many early morning appointments so I don't have to take time off work?)

- What size follicles do you look for before deciding when egg collection should be?

- How many eggs are you trying to get for me at egg collection (given my age, history and test results)?

4. Where do you do egg collection?

- On site or elsewhere?

- Who will do the procedure? You or a colleague? (Most consultants share patients so you won't necessarily have met them before the op.)

- Will I have general anaesthesia or sedation?

- What pain relief will I have after egg collection?

- How long will I need off work after egg collection?

5. When and where is the sperm sample produced?

- Can we see the room beforehand and can my partner do a test sample to check he's comfortable there?

- Can we freeze sperm as a backup? (All clinics should offer this.)

- If so, how much does this cost?

- Can he bring in a sample from home instead?

- When should he do his last ejaculation before THE sample that is to be used?

6. Where is embryo transfer carried out?

- How many days after egg collection do you prefer to do egg transfer? (Most clinics have a preference for two-, three- or five-day transfer – this is properly explained in Chapter 9.)

- What is your view on three-day (eight-cell) transfer versus five-day blastocyst transfer? (Also explained in Chapter 9.)

- What is your policy on single embryo transfer v multiple (for our age and circumstances)?

- What are the risks of a multiple pregnancy?

- How do you grade the embryos? (Some clinics have different grading systems.)

- Will you try to freeze any spare embryos?

7. **How do you rate our chances of success given our age, history and test results?**

   - Is there anything we should do (exercise, acupuncture, diet, supplements, etc.) to increase our chances of a successful IVF cycle with you? (Some clinics advocate acupuncture or total bed rest after transfer, etc.)

8. **What are the risks involved with the procedures (OHSS, etc.) and also any side effects of the drugs?**

9. **In what circumstances would you decide to abandon the cycle?**

   - How common is that and at what stages do things go wrong?

   - If it didn't work, when would we be able to try IVF again and what support would there be from the clinic?

10. **How much does it all cost?**

   - Are the scans/blood tests all included in the base price or are they on top?

   - How much are the drugs on top (given my particular dosage) and what about follow-up consultations (if unsuccessful)?

List of terms

An explanation of common IVF abbreviations and terms (particularly ones used on internet forums)

2WW	Two-week wait	**EC**	egg collection
16dp3dt	16 days past 3-day transfer	**ED**	egg donor
		EDD	estimated due date
AF	Aunt Flo = period arriving/bleeding starting	**ET**	embryo transfer
AH	assisted hatching	**FSH**	follical-stimulating hormone
AHR	assisted human reproduction	**FET**	frozen embryo transfer
AMH	anti-müllerian hormone	**GIFT**	gamete intra-fallopian tube transfer
ART	assisted reproductive technologies	**GS**	gestational surrogate
BBT	basal body temperature	**hCG**	human chorionic gonadotropin
BCP	birth control pill	**HPT**	home pregnancy test
Beta	hCG-level blood test	**ICSI**	intra cytoplasmic sperm injection
BFP/BFN	big fat positive/negative	**IMSI**	intra-cytoplasmic morphologically-selected sperm injection
BMI	body mass index		
COH	controlled ovarian hyperstimulation	**IP**	intended parent
CD	cycle day	**IUI**	intra uterine insemination
DH/DW/DS/DD	dear husband/wife/son/ daughter	**IVF**	in vitro fertilisation

LAP	laparoscopy	**PID**	pelvic inflammatory disease
LMP	last menstrual period		
LH	luteinising hormone	**POAS**	pee on a stick – home pregnancy test
LP	luteal phase		
LPD	luteal phase defect	**POF**	premature ovarian failure
MF	male factor	**PUPO**	pregnant until proven otherwise
NK (cells)	natural killer cells	**TCM**	Traditional Chinese Medicine
OHSS	ovarian hyperstimulation syndrome		
		TSH	thyroid stimulating hormone
PCOS	polycystic ovary syndrome		
		TTC	trying to conceive
PGD	pre implantation genetic diagnosis	**ZIFT**	zygote intra fallopian tube transfer

Acknowledgements

The authors would like to thank:

Everyone at our publisher, Orion, for believing in this book and for their bottomless patience, enthusiasm and for being frighteningly well organised. In particular: Lisa Milton and Amanda Harris, and, in marketing and publicity: Marissa Hussey, Alice Morley and Mark McGinlay. Also a special mention to Jillian Young for her remarkably efficient editorial eyes and for consistently replying to some of the longest and most boring emails in the history of electronic messaging.

Nicola Ibison at James Grant Management for being The Finest Agent In The Northern Hemisphere™. And probably the southern one too. And also for being the single most efficient person we have met and for being particularly effective at kicking Richard's arse, if only metaphorically.

Consultant James Nicopoullos for so generously giving up his time and for checking our facts, adding in his own tips at the end of each chapter and for writing our Foreword.

Gabby Logan for her time and support.

The HFEA press office for being so helpful and for being an invaluable resource for the latest IVF stats.

All the IVF clinics and staff we saw, most notably Liz the lovely sonographer in chapter 14 who handled our miscarriage so sensitively and the experienced sonographer in chapter 15 who stuck her neck out and told us everything would be okay.

Rosie would like to thank: acupuncturist Shereen Kalideen and hypnotherapist Kristin Hayward for keeping her (relatively) sane and healthy throughout the IVF process.

Rosie would also like to thank all of her wonderful friends, especially: Kathryn, Jo and Charmian for their enduring love, wit and wisdom and always knowing the right thing to say; Lucy for her support and general loveliness through every nerve-wracking day of the last round of IVF and the 9 months that followed; Natasha and Beth for graciously understanding the infertility-induced absence during their last pregnancies; Kate for her insight, humour and beautiful photographs of our long-awaited pregnancy; cousins Sarah and Tia for their kindness, sensitivity and advice and all the friends who shared their fertility woes and IVF stories with us, you are a brave and inspiring lot.

Richard would also like to thank all friends, especially: Jools for his tireless patience and generosity in a pub environment, Penny for providing just the right combination of nagging, bullying and threatening language to get me to actually write a book, Caroline for sitting through (and paying for) an enormous number of lunches at which she was forced to listen to endless tales of forced masturbation and sperm (usually mine), Johnny for telling me what IVF was really like before we did it; and finally, the silly friend who told me that he could only get properly aroused in the wank booth when he found an article he'd written in one of the jazz mags. You dirty egotist. You know who you are.

Most importantly we'd like to thank our siblings for their continuing love and support and our parents for being, variously: couriers, taxi drivers, Samaritans, benefactors, advisors and, well, parents.

Finally we'd like to apologise to a border terrier called Jeremy who could not have been prepared for the tsunami of love that would come his way when he entered our lives and, of course, for naming him Jeremy.

Index

AIDS *see* HIV
AMH 65–9, 72, 75–6, 79
Anti-Mullerian Hormone test *see* AMH
ART 88–9
artificial reproduction techniques *see* ART

baby, growth rate of 225
blood tests, commonest *see* fertility
body mass index *see* BMI
BMI 43
Bromocriptine 103

Cabergoline 103
Cetrotide 103
cervical mucus 10
chlamydia, testing for 23, 64, 72, 74
chromosome problems 212
clinics
    basic facts 52
    choosing 42–61
    consultant's view on 60
    cost
        NHS funding 42–4, 51–2, 59
        private 45–6, 52, 58–9, 87, 209
    female view on 42–50
    key factors when deciding 45–9
    male view on 51–9
cost of treatment *see* clinics
Crinone 103
Cyclogest 103

DNA 88, 175, 250
    fragmentation 166, 174
Down's Syndrome test 265, 279
drugs, for IVF 99–114, 183
    buying 106
    chart of common drugs and side-effects
        103
    consultant's view on 114

drugs (*cont.*)
    cost 107
    female view on 99–108
    for first cycle 118
    for Frozen Embryo Transfer 150
    for second cycle 118
    for third cycle 118
    injecting 105, 112–13
        needles 106
    male view on 109–114
    mixing 104–5, 111–12
    side effects 113
    'trigger' 7, 69, 84, 92, 101, 110, 116, 117,
        18, 119, 125, 127, 198
    what they do 99–103, 110

eggs 23, 66–7, 68, 84, 87, 92, *see also* sperm
    collecting 7, 77, 78, 79, 84, 86, 92, 93,
        110, 183
    collection day 93, 116–45, 146, 151, 154
        consultant's view on 143
        female view on 116–25
        ICSI 84, 88–9, 123–4, 146, 154, 156–7,
            158
        male view on 126–43
        post collecting period 93
        risks (OHSS) 118–19, 152, 183
        the facts 117
        the procedure 119–20, 126–7
        'trigger' drug *see* drugs
    donor 89
    fertilise 147
    maturing 101–2, 110
    production 126
    sharing 89
    stimulation 7
    the facts 107
embryo 7, 23, 87, 147, 158–9
    affected by scent 169, 171

embryo (*cont.*)
  arrested 146
  blastocoel 146
  blastocysts 85, 146, 148, 149–50, 155,
      180, 181
  compacting 149
  divide 147–8, 155
  donor 89
  failure to develop, reasons why 212
  fragmentation 146
  Frozen Embryo Transfer (FET) 150
  implant 7, 93, 148
  inner cell mass 146
  making 84–5, 93
  morula 146, 181
  putting in womb 85–6
  terminology 146
  timeline 180–1
  transfer of 162–77
    consultant's view on 176
    female view on 162–9
    male view on 170–76
    pregnancy rate for no. and stage of
        embryos
    transferred 165–9
    single embryo transfer, pros/cons 164
    the procedure 164–5, 170–6
  trophectoderm 146

fallopian tubes 23, 24
fertilisation results 145–61
  consultant's view on 160
  embryo terminology 146
  female view on 145–53
  male view on 154–59
  timeline 146–50, 154–6
fertility
  facts 10
  help, and seeing GP 22
  low 67–72
  tests 22–41
    AMH levels 65–9, 72, 75–6, 79
    commonest blood 23
    consultant's view on 40
    female view on 22–7
    male view on 28–40
fertility monitor 11–12
follicle-stimulating hormone *see* FSH
follicles 23, 84, 87, 88, 116, 118, 183
Frozen Embryo Transfer (FET) 150
FSH 23, 25, 40, 43, 66, 103

German measles 23
Gestone 103

Gonal-F 103
Goserelin 103

Harmony Test 265
HCG *see* Human Chorionic Gonadotropin
hepatitis, testing for 43, 64, 74
HFEA *see* Human Fertilisation and
        Embryology Authority
HIV, testing for 43, 64–5, 74
home pregnancy test *see* pregnancy kits
hormone drugs 99–101
hormones 23, *see also* FSH, LH
HPT *see* pregnancy kits
HSG *see* hysterosalpingogram
Human Chorionic Gonadotropin 46, 101,
        106, 181, 195, 198, 201
Human Fertilisation and Embryology
        Authority 9, 52, 164
hypnotherapy 11–12, 14
hysterosalpingogram 24
hysteroscopy 24

ICSI *see* eggs
IMSI 89, 146, 154
infertility 8–9
  attempts to conceive
    consultant's view on 20
    female view on 8–14
    male view on 15–20
  definition 9
  fertility show at Olympia 54–8
  main causes of in UK 25
  reasons for, possible 17
  tests, *see also* fertility tests
    consultant's view on 40
    female, for 22–7
    male, for 23, 28–40, 48
  unexplained reasons for 25–6
IUI 88
IVF 146, 154, *see also* drugs, pregnancy
  appointment 62–80
    consultant's view on 80
    extra tests 64–9, 74
    female view on 62–72
    male view on 73–9
    preliminary questions asked 63–4, 73
    questions to ask consultant 69, 78,
        293–5
  attempts 271
  chance of success 87
  consultation, first 82–97
    artificial reproductive options 88–9
    consultant's view on 97
    female view on 82–91

consultation (cont.)
  male view on 92–7
    egg collection day 93, see also eggs
    post egg collection period 93
  lessons learnt from 281–92
    consultant's view on 291
    female view on 282–8
    male view on 289–91
  national live birth rate per cycle 47
  percentage of UK babies born, conceived
    through 1
  process of 7, 84–6, 92
    complications 87
    cost 58, 59, 87, 209, see also clinics
    making embryos 84–5
    putting embryos in womb 85–6
    the wait 86–7
  timeline 237–9
  stages of 290–1
  successful 259–80
    consultant's view on 279
    female view on 259–69
    male view on 270–79
  UK couples undergoing treatment 1

laparoscopy 24
LH 23, 25, 40, 66, 103
luteinizing hormone see LH

Menogon 103
Menopur 103
menstrual cycle 23, 66, 103, 190
Merional 103
miscarriages 235–58
  consultant's view on 257
  female view on 235–46
  male view on 247–56
  recovery from 244
  surviving a 245–6
  the facts 236, 240, 243
  timeline leading to 237–9
  types of 245
morning sickness 277

Nafarelin buserelin 103

oestradiol 23
oestrogen 23
OHSS 118–19, 152, 183
orgalutran-gonadotropin-releasing
  hormone 103
Ovarian Hyperstimulation Syndrome 117,
  118

ovaries 23, 24, 45, 66, 68, 100, 103, 110,
  116, 119, 120, 151, 152, 183, 190
Ovitrelle 101, 118, 119
ovulation 10, 11, 12, 14, 20, 23, 46, 66, 84,
  92, 107, 190, 290
  problems 25
  stimulating 100, 103, 110
  switching off 7, 84, 92, 100–1, 103, 110

pelvic ultrasound scan 24
pituitary gland 23
pregnancy, see also IVF
  kits 179, 181, 194, 201–2, see also Human
    Chorionic Gonadotropin
    choice of 196
    dos and don'ts 198
    using 203
  morning sickness 277
  negative results 208–19
    consultant's view on 219
    female view on 208–13
    male view on 214–18
    possible causes 212
  positive results 221–33
    consultant's view on 233
    continuing success rates 225
    Down's Syndrome test 265, 279
    female view on 221–6
    growth rate of baby 225
    male view on 227–32
    scans 24, 45, 58, 70, 71, 87, 100, 101,
      116, 117, 119, 143, 205, 223–4,
      225, 229–30, 233, 237, 244, 264,
      265, 266, 267, 269, 270, 272–4,
      291, 293, 295
    4D 276, 279
    4 weeks 230
    6 weeks 233
    7 weeks 7, 223, 230, 235, 248, 250,
      263, 272
    8 weeks 233
    9 weeks 263, 271, 272
    10 weeks 7, 230, 238
    12 weeks 7, 168, 228, 231, 232, 233,
      264, 265, 274, 279
    16 weeks 231
    20 weeks 231, 266, 267, 278, 291
    26–30 weeks 231
    40 weeks 231
    pelvic ultrasound 24
    timing of 230–2
  rate for no. and stage of embryos
    transferred 165–9
  success rates 9, 13

pregnancy (*cont.*)
  test, day of the 194–207
    consultant's view 206
    female view on 194–200
    male view on 201–6
    timing of 195–6
  testing 180, 290
    delaying testing 180, 186, 191, 192
Pregnant Until Proven Otherwise *see* PUPO
Pregnyl 113
progesterone 23, 25, 86, 102, 110, 182,
        183–4, 185, 189
  and side effects 102, 103, 183
  what it does 190
Progynova 103
pronuclei 147
PUPO 179
puregon luteinizing hormone *see* LH

Rubella *see* German measles

scans *see* pregnancy
sex 12, 14
  male view on 15–16
  reasons for avoiding 16
sperm 40, 88, 93, 97, 147
  donor 89

sperm (*cont.*)
  facts 30
  female 10
  freezing 74–5, 78, 97, 141, 142
  male 10, 12
  optimum 31
  samples 78, 28–40, 78, 124–5
    'incident in the booth' 130–42
  test 23
  understanding test report 38
stress relief 14

temperature, body 10, 11–12
trophectoderm 146
two-week wait 178–93
  consultant's view on 192
  female view on 178–86
  male view on 187–92
    on female response 187–92

uterus 24

vitamins 11–12

womb lining 23
  thickening 102

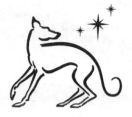